AGING ISSUES, HEALTH AND FINANCIAL ALTERNATIVES

ALZHEIMER'S DISEASE

A CAREGIVERS GUIDE

Aging Issues, Health and Financial Alternatives

Additional books in this series can be found on Nova's website under the Series tab.

Additional e-books in this series can be found on Nova's website under the e-book tab.

AGING ISSUES, HEALTH AND FINANCIAL ALTERNATIVES

ALZHEIMER'S DISEASE

A CAREGIVERS GUIDE

DIANA B. WATKINS
EDITOR

NOVA BIOMEDICAL

New York

For permission to use material from this book please contact us:
Telephone 631-231-7269; Fax 631-231-8175
Web Site: http://www.novapublishers.com

Library of Congress Cataloging-in-Publication Data

ISBN: 978-1-63117-720-0

Published by Nova Science Publishers, Inc. † New York

CONTENTS

PREFACE

Alzheimer's disease is an illness of the brain. It causes large numbers of nerve cells in the brain to die. This affects a person's ability to remember things and think clearly. People with AD become forgetful and easily confused. They may have a hard time concentrating and behave in odd ways. These problems get worse as the illness gets worse, making it more difficult for caregivers. Caring for a person with Alzheimer's disease is a challenge that calls upon the patience, creativity, knowledge, and skills of each caregiver. This book is for those who provide in-home care for people with Alzheimer's disease or related disorders. The goal is to improve home safety by identifying potential problems in the home and offering possible solutions to help prevent accidents.

Chapter 1 - This chapter is for people who care for family members or others with Alzheimer's disease (AD) at home. AD is an illness that changes the brain. It causes people to lose the ability to remember, think, and use good judgment and to have trouble taking care of themselves. Over time, as the disease gets worse, they will need more help.

Sometimes, taking care of the person with AD makes you feel good because you are providing love and comfort. Other times, it can be overwhelming. Also, each day brings new challenges. You may not even realize how much you have taken on because the changes can happen slowly over a long period of time.

The authors have written this chapter to help you learn about and cope with these changes and challenges. You will find suggestions for taking care of yourself, which helps you to be a good caregiver.

The information in this chapter comes from other caregivers and from medical research, such as that funded by the National Institute on Aging

(NIA). NIA is part of the National Institutes of Health, the nation's medical research agency. NIA leads the federal effort to find the cause of and treatment for Alzheimer's disease.

The chapter tells you how to:

- Understand how AD changes a person
- Learn how to cope with these changes
- Help family and friends understand AD
- Plan for the future
- Make your home safe for the person with AD
- Manage everyday activities like eating, bathing, dressing, and grooming
- Take care of yourself
- Get help with caregiving
- Find out about helpful resources, such as websites, support groups, government agencies, and adult day care programs
- Choose a full-time care facility for the person with AD if needed
- Learn about common behavior and medical problems of people with AD and some medicines that may help
- Cope with late-stage AD

This chapter contains a lot of information. Please don't feel that you have to read it all at one time. You can use the tools provided to find what you need quickly.

Chapter 2 - Caring for a person with Alzheimer's disease is a challenge that calls upon the patience, creativity, knowledge, and skills of each caregiver. The authors hope that this chapter will help you cope with some of these challenges and develop creative solutions to increase the security and freedom of the person with Alzheimer's in your home, as well as your own peace of mind.

This chapter is for those who provide in-home care for people with Alzheimer's disease or related disorders. The authors' goal is to improve home safety by identifying potential problems in the home and offering possible solutions to help prevent accidents.

The authors begin with a checklist to help you make each room in your home a safer environment for the person with Alzheimer's. Next, the authors hope to increase awareness of the ways specific impairments associated with the disease can create particular safety hazards in the home. Home safety tips are listed to help you cope with some of the more hazardous behaviors that may occur as the disease advances. The authors also include tips for managing driving and planning for natural disaster safety. The chapter ends with a list of resources for family caregivers.

In: Alzheimer's Disease: A Caregivers Guide ISBN: 978-1-63117-720-0
Editor: Diana B. Watkins

Chapter 1

CARING FOR A PERSON WITH ALZHEIMER'S DISEASE: YOUR EASY-TO-USE GUIDE FROM THE NATIONAL INSTITUTE ON AGING*

National Institute of Aging

ABOUT THIS CHAPTER

This chapter is for people who care for family members or others with Alzheimer's disease (AD) at home. AD is an illness that changes the brain. It causes people to lose the ability to remember, think, and use good judgment and to have trouble taking care of themselves. Over time, as the disease gets worse, they will need more help.

Sometimes, taking care of the person with AD makes you feel good because you are providing love and comfort. Other times, it can be overwhelming. Also, each day brings new challenges. You may not even realize how much you have taken on because the changes can happen slowly over a long period of time.

We've written this chapter to help you learn about and cope with these changes and challenges. You will find suggestions for taking care of yourself, which helps you to be a good caregiver.

---

* This is an edited, reformatted and augmented version of NIH Publication No. 12-6173, updated May 2013.

The information in this chapter comes from other caregivers and from medical research, such as that funded by the National Institute on Aging (NIA). NIA is part of the National Institutes of Health, the nation's medical research agency. NIA leads the federal effort to find the cause of and treatment for Alzheimer's disease.

The chapter tells you how to:

- Understand how AD changes a person
- Learn how to cope with these changes
- Help family and friends understand AD
- Plan for the future
- Make your home safe for the person with AD
- Manage everyday activities like eating, bathing, dressing, and grooming
- Take care of yourself
- Get help with caregiving
- Find out about helpful resources, such as websites, support groups, government agencies, and adult day care programs
- Choose a full-time care facility for the person with AD if needed
- Learn about common behavior and medical problems of people with AD and some medicines that may help
- Cope with late-stage AD

This chapter contains a lot of information. Please don't feel that you have to read it all at one time. You can use the tools listed below to find what you need quickly.

UNDERSTANDING AD

Sometimes, you may feel that you don't know how to care for the person with AD. You're not alone. Each day may bring different challenges. Learning about AD can help you understand and cope with these challenges. Below, we discuss the stages of AD and tell you how to learn more about the illness.

Stages of AD and What They Mean

Alzheimer's disease consists of three main stages: mild (sometimes called early-stage), moderate, and severe (sometimes called late-stage). Understanding these stages can help you plan ahead.

Mild Alzheimer's disease. In mild AD, the first stage, people often have some memory loss and small changes in their personality. They may forget recent events or the names of familiar people or things. They may no longer be able to solve simple math problems. People with mild AD also slowly lose the ability to plan and organize. For example, they may have trouble making a grocery list and finding items in the store.

Moderate Alzheimer's disease. This is the middle stage of AD. Memory loss and confusion become more obvious. People have more trouble organizing, planning, and following instructions. They may need help getting dressed and may start having problems with incontinence. This means they can't control their bladder and/or bowels. People with moderate-stage AD may have trouble recognizing family members and friends. They may not know where they are or what day or year it is. They also may lack judgment and begin to wander, so people with moderate AD should not be left alone. They may become restless and begin repeating movements late in the day. Also, they may have trouble sleeping. Personality changes can become more serious. People with moderate AD may make threats, accuse others of stealing, curse, kick, hit, bite, scream, or grab things.

Severe Alzheimer's disease. This is the last stage of Alzheimer's and ends in the death of the person. Severe AD is sometimes called late-stage AD. In this stage, people often need help with all their daily needs. They may not be able to walk or sit up without help. They may not be able to talk and often cannot recognize family members. They may have trouble swallowing and refuse to eat.

How to Learn More about AD

Here are some ways to help you learn more about AD:

- Talk with a doctor or other health care provider about AD. Ask your doctor to refer you to someone who specializes in AD.
- Ask your doctor or AD specialist about good sources of information.
- Check out books, CDs, DVDs, or videos on AD from the library.
- Go to educational programs and workshops on AD.
- Visit websites on AD such as www.alzheimers.gov, www.nia.nih.gov/alzheimers, or www.alz.org. Use search engines to find more information.
- Talk about AD with friends and family to get advice and support.
- Try to find a support group for caregivers. You want a group in which the caregivers are taking care of someone who is in the same stage of AD as the person you are caring for. Also, you may be able to find an Internet-based support group. This is helpful for some caregivers, because it means they don't have to leave home to be a part of the group. The Alzheimer's Association (www.alz.org) is a good resource to help find support groups.

Caring for a Person with AD

Understanding How AD Changes People— Challenges and Coping Strategies

Alzheimer's disease is an illness of the brain. It causes large numbers of nerve cells in the brain to die. This affects a person's ability to remember things and think clearly. People with AD become forgetful and easily confused. They may have a hard time concentrating and behave in odd ways. These problems get worse as the illness gets worse, making your job as caregiver harder.

It's important to remember that the disease, not the person with AD, causes these changes. Also, each person with AD may not have all the problems we talk about in this book.

The following sections describe the three main challenges that you may face as you care for someone with AD:

1. changes in communication skills
2. changes in personality and behavior
3. changes in intimacy and sexuality

Each section includes information on how to cope with these challenges.

1. Challenge: changes in communication skills

Communication is hard for people with AD because they have trouble remembering things. They may struggle to find words or forget what they want to say. You may feel impatient and wish they could just say what they want, but they can't. It may help you to know more about common communication problems caused by AD. Once you know more, you'll have a better sense of how to cope.

Here are some communication problems caused by AD:

- Trouble finding the right word when speaking
- Problems understanding what words mean
- Problems paying attention during long conversations
- Loss of train-of-thought when talking
- Trouble remembering the steps in common activities, such as cooking a meal, paying bills, getting dressed, or doing laundry
- Problems blocking out background noises from the radio, TV, telephone calls, or conversations in the room
- Frustration if communication isn't working
- Being very sensitive to touch and to the tone and loudness of voices

Also, AD causes some people to get confused about language. For example, the person might forget or no longer understand English if it was learned as a second language. Instead, he or she might understand and use only the first language learned, such as Spanish.

How to cope with changes in communication skills

The first step is to understand that the disease causes changes in these skills. The second step is to try some tips that may make communication easier. For example, keep the following suggestions in mind as you go about day-to-day care.

To connect with a person who has AD:

- Make eye contact to get his or her attention, and call the person by name.
- Be aware of your tone and how loud your voice is, how you look at the person, and your "body language." Body language is the message you send just by the way you hold your body. For example, if you stand with your arms folded very tightly, you may send a message that you are tense or angry.
- Encourage a two-way conversation for as long as possible. This helps the person with AD feel better about himself or herself.
- Use other methods besides speaking to help the person, such as gentle touching to guide him or her.
- Try distracting someone with AD if communication creates problems. For example, offer a fun activity such as a snack or a walk around the neighborhood.

To encourage the person with AD to communicate with you:

- Show a warm, loving, matter-of-fact manner.
- Hold the person's hand while you talk.
- Be open to the person's concerns, even if he or she is hard to understand.
- Let him or her make some decisions and stay involved.
- Be patient with angry outbursts. Remember, it's the illness "talking."
- If you become frustrated, take a "timeout" for yourself.

To speak effectively with a person who has AD:

- Offer simple, step-by-step instructions.
- Repeat instructions and allow more time for a response. Try not to interrupt.
- Don't talk about the person as if he or she isn't there.
- Don't talk to the person using "baby talk" or a "baby voice."

Here are some examples of what you can say:

- "Let's try this way," instead of pointing out mistakes
- "Please do this," instead of "Don't do this"
- "Thanks for helping," even if the results aren't perfect

Helping a Person Who Is Aware of Memory Loss

AD is being diagnosed at earlier stages. This means that many people are aware of how the disease is affecting their memory. Here are tips on how to help someone who knows that he or she has memory problems:

- Take time to listen. The person may want to talk about the changes he or she is noticing.
- Be as sensitive as you can. Don't just correct the person every time he or she forgets something or says something odd. Try to understand that it's a struggle for the person to communicate.
- Be patient when someone with AD has trouble finding the right words or putting feelings into words.
- Help the person find words to express thoughts and feelings.
  For example, Mrs. D cried after forgetting her garden club meeting. She finally said, "I wish they stopped." Her daughter said, "You wish your friends had stopped by for you." Mrs. D nodded and repeated some of the words. Then Mrs. D said, "I want to go." Her daughter said, "You want to go to the garden club meeting." Again, Mrs. D nodded and repeated the words.
- Be careful not to put words in the person's mouth or "fill in the blanks" too quickly.
- As people lose the ability to talk clearly, they may rely on other ways to communicate their thoughts and feelings.
  For example, their facial expressions may show sadness, anger, or frustration. Grasping at their undergarments may tell you they need to use the bathroom.

You also can:

- Ask questions that require a yes or no answer. For example, you could say, "Are you tired?" instead of "How do you feel?"

- Limit the number of choices. For example, you could say, "Would you like a hamburger or chicken for dinner?" instead of "What would you like for dinner?"
- Use different words if he or she doesn't understand what you say the first time. For example, if you ask the person whether he or she is hungry and you don't get a response, you could say, "Dinner is ready now. Let's eat."
- Try not to say, "Don't you remember?" or "I told you."

2. Challenge: changes in personality and behavior

Because AD causes brain cells to die, the brain works less well over time. This changes how a person acts. You will notice that he or she will have good days and bad days.

Here are some common personality changes you may see:

- Getting upset, worried, and angry more easily
- Acting depressed or not interested in things
- Hiding things or believing other people are hiding things
- Imagining things that aren't there
- Wandering away from home
- Pacing a lot of the time
- Showing unusual sexual behavior
- Hitting you or other people
- Misunderstanding what he or she sees or hears

Also, you may notice that the person stops caring about how he or she looks, stops bathing, and wants to wear the same clothes every day.

CHANGES IN BEHAVIOR

You may see changes in behavior that the disease didn't cause. For example, certain medicines, severe pain, poor eyesight or hearing, and fatigue can cause behavior changes. If you don't know what is causing the problem, call the doctor.

Other factors that may affect how people with AD behave

In addition to changes in the brain, the following things may affect how people with AD behave.

How they feel:

- Sadness, fear, or a feeling of being overwhelmed
- Stress caused by something or someone
- Confusion after a change in routine, including travel
- Anxiety about going to a certain place

Health-related problems:

- Illness or pain
- New medications
- Lack of sleep
- Infections, constipation, hunger, or thirst
- Poor eyesight or hearing
- Alcohol abuse
- Too much caffeine

Problems in their surroundings:

- Being in a place he or she doesn't know well.
- Too much noise, such as TV, radio, or many people talking at once. Noise can cause confusion or frustration.
- Stepping from one type of flooring to another. The change in texture or the way the floor looks may make the person think he or she needs to take a step down.
- Misunderstanding signs. Some signs may cause confusion. For example, one person with AD thought a sign reading "Wet Floor" meant he should urinate on the floor.
- Mirrors. Someone with AD may think that a mirror image is another person in the room.

How to cope with personality and behavior changes

Here are some ways to cope with changes in personality and behavior:

- Keep things simple. Ask or say one thing at a time.
- Have a daily routine, so the person knows when certain things will happen.
- Reassure the person that he or she is safe and you are there to help.
- Focus on his or her feelings rather than words. For example, say, "You seem worried."
- Don't argue or try to reason with the person.
- Try not to show your anger or frustration. Step back. Take deep breaths, and count to 10. If safe, leave the room for a few minutes.
- Use humor when you can.
- Give people who pace a lot a safe place to walk. Provide comfortable, sturdy shoes. Give them light snacks to eat as they walk, so they don't lose too much weight, and make sure they have enough to drink.

Use distractions:

- Try using music, singing, or dancing to distract the person. One caregiver found that giving her husband chewing gum stopped his cursing.
- Ask for help. For instance, say, "Let's set the table" or "I really need help folding the clothes."

Other ideas:

- Enroll the person in the MedicAlert®+Alzheimer's Association Safe Return® Program. If people with AD wander away from home, this program can help get them home safely (www.alz.org).
- Talk to the doctor about any serious behavior or emotional problems, such as hitting, biting, depression, or hallucinations.

How to cope with sleep problems

Evenings are hard for many people with AD. Some may become restless or irritable around dinnertime. This restlessness is called "sundowning." It may even be hard to get the person to go to bed and stay there.

Here are some tips that may help:

- Help the person get exercise each day, limit naps, and make sure the person gets enough rest at night. Being overly tired can increase late-afternoon and nighttime restlessness.
- Plan activities that use more energy early in the day. For example, try bathing in the morning or having the largest family meal in the middle of the day.
- Set a quiet, peaceful mood in the evening to help the person relax. Keep the lights low, try to reduce the noise levels, and play soothing music if he or she enjoys it.
- Try to have the person go to bed at the same time each night. A bedtime routine, such as reading out loud, also may help.
- Limit caffeine.
- Use nightlights in the bedroom, hall, and bathroom.

How to cope with hallucinations and delusions

As the disease progresses, the person with AD may have hallucinations. During a hallucination, a person sees, hears, smells, tastes, or feels something that isn't there. For example, the person may see his or her dead mother in the room. He or she also may have delusions. Delusions are false beliefs that the person thinks are real. For example, the person may think his or her spouse is in love with someone else.

Here are some things you can do:

- Tell the doctor or AD specialist about the delusions or hallucinations.
- Discuss with the doctor any illnesses the person has and medicines he or she is taking. Sometimes an illness or medicine may cause hallucinations or delusions.
- Try not to argue about what the person with AD sees or hears. Comfort the person if he or she is afraid.
- Distract the person. Sometimes moving to another room or going outside for a walk helps.
- Turn off the TV when violent or upsetting programs are on. Someone with AD may think these events are really going on in the room.
- Make sure the person is safe and can't reach anything that could be used to hurt anyone or him or herself.

How to cope with paranoia

Paranoia is a type of delusion in which a person may believe— without a good reason—that others are mean, lying, unfair, or "out to get him or her." He or she may become suspicious, fearful, or jealous of people.

In a person with AD, paranoia often is linked to memory loss. It can become worse as memory loss gets worse. For example, the person may become paranoid if he or she forgets:

- Where he or she put something. The person may believe that someone is taking his or her things.
- That you are the person's caregiver. Someone with AD might not trust you if he or she thinks you are a stranger.
- People to whom he or she has been introduced. The person may believe that strangers will be harmful.
- Directions you just gave. The person may think you are trying to trick him or her.

Paranoia may be the person's way of expressing loss. The person may blame or accuse others because no other explanation seems to make sense.

Here are some tips for dealing with paranoia:

- Try not to react if the person blames you for something.
- Don't argue with him or her.
- Let the person know that he or she is safe.
- Use gentle touching or hugging to show the person you care.
- Explain to others that the person is acting this way because he or she has AD.
- Search for missing things to distract the person; then talk about what you found. For example, talk about a photograph or keepsake.
- Have extra sets of keys or eyeglasses in case they are lost.

CHECK IT OUT!

Someone with AD may have a good reason for acting a certain way. He or she may not be paranoid. There are people who take advantage of weak and elderly people. Find out if someone is trying to abuse or steal from the person with AD.

How to cope with agitation and aggression

Agitation means that a person is restless and worried. He or she doesn't seem to be able to settle down. Agitated people may pace a lot, not be able to sleep, or act aggressively toward others. They may verbally lash out or try to hit or hurt someone. When this happens, try to find the cause. There is usually a reason.

For example, the person may have:

- Pain, depression, or stress
- Too little rest or sleep
- Constipation
- Soiled underwear or diaper

Here are some other causes of agitation and aggression:

- Sudden change in a well-known place, routine, or person
- A feeling of loss—for example, the person with AD may miss driving or caring for children
- Too much noise or confusion or too many people around
- Being pushed by others to do something—for example, to bathe or remember events or people—when AD has made the activity very hard or impossible
- Feeling lonely and not having enough contact with other people
- Interaction of medicines

Here are suggestions to help you cope with agitation and aggression:

- Look for the early signs of agitation or aggression. Then you can deal with the cause before the problem behaviors start.
- Doing nothing can make things worse. Try to find the causes of the behavior. If you deal with the causes, the behavior may stop.
- Slow down and try to relax if you think your own worries may be affecting the person with AD. Try to find a way to take a break from caregiving.
- Allow the person to keep as much control in his or her life as possible.
- Try to distract the person with a favorite snack, object, or activity.

You also can:

- Reassure him or her. Speak calmly. Listen to the person's concerns and frustrations. Try to show that you understand if the person is angry or fearful.
- Keep well-loved objects and photographs around the house. This can make the person feel more secure.
- Reduce noise, clutter, or the number of people in the room.
- Try gentle touching, soothing music, reading, or walks.
- Build quiet times into the day, along with activities.
- Limit the amount of caffeine, sugar, and "junk food" the person drinks and eats.

Here are things the doctor can do:

- Give the person a medical exam to find any problems that may cause the behavior. These problems might include pain, depression, or the effects of certain medicines.
- Check the person's vision and hearing each year.

Here are some important things to do when the person is aggressive:

- Protect yourself and your family members from aggressive behavior. If you have to, stay at a safe distance from the person until the behavior stops.
- As much as possible, protect the person from hurting himself or herself.
- Ask the doctor or AD specialist if medicine may be needed to prevent or reduce agitation or aggression.

How to cope with wandering

Many people with AD wander away from their home or caregiver. As the caregiver, you need to know how to limit wandering and prevent the person from becoming lost. This will help keep the person safe and give you greater peace of mind.

KEEP TO A ROUTINE

Try to keep to a routine, such as bathing, dressing, and eating at the same time each day.

Coping with changes is hard for someone with AD.

Try to follow these tips before the person with AD wanders:

- Make sure the person carries some kind of ID or wears a medical bracelet. If the person gets lost, an ID will let others know about his or her illness. It also shows where the person lives.
- Consider enrolling the person in the MedicAlert®+ Alzheimer's Association Safe Return® Program (see www.alz.org or call 1-888-572-8566 to find the program in your area). This service is not affiliated with the National Institute on Aging. There may be a charge for this service.
- Let neighbors and the local police know that the person with AD tends to wander.
- Keep a recent photograph or video recording of the person to help police if the person becomes lost.
- Keep doors locked. Consider a keyed deadbolt, or add another lock placed up high or down low on the door. If the person can open a lock, you may need to get a new latch or lock.
- Install an "announcing system" that chimes when the door opens.

How to cope with rummaging and hiding things

Someone with AD may start rummaging or searching through cabinets, drawers, closets, the refrigerator, and other places where things are stored. He or she also may hide items around the house. This behavior can be annoying or even dangerous for the caregiver or family members. If you get angry, try to remember that this behavior is part of the disease.

In some cases, there might be a logical reason for this behavior. For instance, the person may be looking for something specific, although he or she may not be able to tell you what it is. He or she may be hungry or bored. Try to understand what is causing the behavior so you can fit your response to the cause.

Here are some other steps to take:

- Lock up dangerous or toxic products, or place them out of the person's sight and reach.
- Remove spoiled food from the refrigerator and cabinets. Someone with AD may look for snacks, but lack the judgment or sense of taste to stay away from spoiled foods.
- Remove valuable items that could be misplaced or hidden by the person, like important papers, checkbooks, charge cards, jewelry, and keys.
- People with AD often hide, lose, or throw away mail. If this is a serious problem, consider getting a post office box. If you have a yard with a fence and a locked gate, place your mailbox outside the gate.
- Keep the person with AD from going into unused rooms. This limits his or her rummaging through and hiding things.
- Search the house to learn where the person often hides things. Once you find these places, check them often, out of sight of the person.
- Keep all trash cans covered or out of sight. People with AD may not remember the purpose of the container or may rummage through it.
- Check trash containers before you empty them, in case something has been hidden there or thrown away by accident.

You also can create a special place where the person with AD can rummage freely or sort things. This could be a chest of drawers, a bag of objects, or a basket of clothing to fold or unfold. Give him or her a personal box, chest, or cupboard to store special objects. You may have to remind the person where to find his or her personal storage place.

3. Challenge: changes in intimacy and sexuality

Intimacy is the special bond we share with a person we love and respect. It includes the way we talk and act toward one another. This bond can exist between spouses or partners, family members, and friends. AD often changes the intimacy between people.

Sexuality is one type of intimacy. It is an important way that spouses or partners express their feelings physically for one another.

AD can cause changes in intimacy and sexuality in both the person with AD and the caregiver. The person with AD may be stressed by the changes in his or her memory and behaviors. Fear, worry, depression, anger, and low self-esteem (how much the person likes himself or herself) are common. The person may become dependent and cling to you. He or she may not remember your life together and feelings toward one another. Sometimes the person may even fall in love with someone else.

You, the caregiver, may pull away from the person in both an emotional and physical sense. You may be upset by the demands of caregiving. You also may feel frustrated by the person's constant forgetfulness, repeated questions, and other bothersome behaviors.

Most caregivers learn how to cope with these challenges, but it takes time. Some learn to live with the illness and find new meaning in their relationships with people who have AD.

How to cope with changes in intimacy

Remember that most people with AD need to feel that someone loves and cares about them. They also need to spend time with other people as well as you. Your efforts to take care of these needs can help the person with AD to feel happy and safe.

It's important to reassure the person that:

- You love him or her
- You will keep him or her safe
- Others also care about him or her

When intimacy changes, the following tips may help you cope with your own needs:

- Talk with a doctor, social worker, or clergy member about these changes. It may feel awkward to talk about such personal issues, but it can help.
- Talk about your concerns in a support group.
- Think more about the positive parts of the relationship.

- Get more information. Some books, articles, and DVDs/videos can help you understand how AD affects intimacy. For help finding resources, check the websites or call the phone numbers of the organizations listed in this book.

HYPERSEXUALITY

Sometimes, people with AD are overly interested in sex. This is called "hypersexuality." The person may masturbate a lot and try to seduce others. These behaviors are symptoms of the disease and don't always mean that the person wants to have sex.

To cope with hypersexuality, try giving the person more attention and reassurance. You might gently touch, hug, or use other kinds of affection to meet his or her emotional needs. Some people with this problem need medicine to control their behaviors. Talk to the doctor about what steps to take.

How to cope with changes in sexuality

The well spouse/partner or the person with AD may lose interest in having sex. This change can make you feel lonely or frustrated. Here are some possible reasons for changes in sexual interest.

The well spouse/partner may feel that:

- It's not okay to have sex with someone who has AD
- The person with AD seems like a stranger
- The person with AD seems to forget that the spouse/partner is there or how to make love

A person with AD may have:

- Side effects from medications that affect his or her sexual interest
- Memory loss, changes in the brain, or depression that affects his or her interest in sex

Here are some suggestions for coping with changes in sexuality:

- Explore new ways of spending time together.

- Focus on other ways to show affection. Some caregivers find that snuggling or holding hands reduces their need for a sexual relationship.
- Focus on other ways to show affection.
- Try other nonsexual forms of touching, such as giving a massage, hugging, and dancing.
- Consider other ways to meet your sexual needs. Some caregivers report that they masturbate to meet their needs.

Helping Family Members and Others Understand AD

Deciding when and how to tell family members and friends

When you learn that someone you love has AD, you may wonder when and how to tell your family and friends. You may be worried about how others will react to or treat the person. While there is no single right way to tell others, we've listed some things to think about.

Think about the following questions:

- Are others already wondering what is going on?
- Do you want to keep this information to yourself?
- Are you embarrassed?
- Do you want to tell others so that you can get support from family members and friends?
- Are you afraid that you will burden others?
- Does keeping this information secret take too much of your energy?
- Are you afraid others won't understand?

Realize that family and friends often sense that something is wrong before they are told. AD is hard to keep secret. When the time seems right, it is best for you to be honest with family, friends, and others. Use this as a chance to educate them about AD.

For example, you can:

- Tell them about the disease and its effects.

- Share books and information to help them understand what you and the person with AD are going through.
- Tell them how they can learn more.
- Tell them what they can do to help. Let them know you need breaks.

Help family and friends understand how to interact with the person who has AD. You can:

- Help them realize what the person still can do and how much he or she still can understand.
- Give them suggestions about how to start talking with the person. For example, "Hello George, I'm John. We used to work together."
- Help them avoid correcting the person with AD if he or she makes a mistake or forgets something.
- Help them plan fun activities with the person, such as going to family reunions; church, temple, or mosque gatherings; other community activities; or visiting old friends.

Communicate with others when you're out in public. Some caregivers carry a card that explains why the person with AD might say or do odd things. For example, the card could read, "My family member has Alzheimer's disease. He or she might say or do things that are unexpected. Thank you for your understanding."

The card allows you to let others know about the person's AD without the person hearing you. It also means that you don't have to keep explaining things.

Helping children understand AD

When a family member has AD, it affects everyone in the family, including children and grandchildren. It's important to talk to them about what is happening. How much and what kind of information you share depends on the child's age. It also depends on his or her relationship to the person with AD.

Give children information about AD that they can understand. There are good books about AD for children of all ages. Some are listed on the Alzheimer's Disease Education and Referral (ADEAR) Center website, www.nia.nih.gov/alzheimers.

Here are some other suggestions to help children understand what is happening:

- Answer their questions simply and honestly. For example, you might tell a young child, "Grandma has an illness that makes it hard for her to remember things."
- Help them know that their feelings of sadness and anger are normal.
- Comfort them. Tell them no one caused the disease. Young children may think they did something to hurt their grandparent.

If the child lives in the same house as someone with AD:

- Don't expect a young child to help take care of or "babysit" the person with AD.
- Make sure the child has time for his or her own interests and needs, such as playing with friends, going to school activities, or doing homework.
- Make sure you spend time with your child, so he or she doesn't feel that all your attention is on the person with AD.
- Help the child understand your feelings. Be honest about your feelings when you talk with a child, but don't overwhelm him or her.

Many younger children will look to you to see how to act around the person with AD. Show children they can still talk with the person, and help them enjoy things each day. Doing fun things together can help both the child and the person with AD.

Here are some things they might do:

- Do simple arts and crafts.
- Play music.
- Sing.
- Look through photo albums.
- Read stories out loud.

Some children may not talk about their negative feelings, but you may see changes in how they act. Problems at school, with friends, or at home can be a sign that they are upset. You may want to ask a school counselor or a social worker to help your child understand what is happening and learn how to cope. Be sure to check with your child often to see how he or she is feeling.

A teenager might find it very hard to accept how the person with AD has changed. He or she may find the changes upsetting or embarrassing and not want to be around the person. It's a good idea to talk with teenagers about their concerns and feelings. Don't force them to spend time with the person who has AD. This could make things worse.

If the stress of living with someone who has AD becomes too great for a child, think about placing the person with AD into a respite care facility. Then, both you and your child can get a much-needed break.

Planning Ahead—Health, Legal, and Financial Issues

When someone is diagnosed with AD, you need to start getting his or her health, legal, and financial affairs in order. You want to plan for the future, if possible, with help from the person while he or she can still make decisions. You need to review all of his or her health, legal, and financial information to make sure it reflects the person's wishes.

Update health care, legal, and financial information

Check to see that you have the following documents and that they are up to date:

- Durable Power of Attorney for Finances gives someone called a trustee the power to make legal and financial decisions for the person with AD
- Durable Power of Attorney for Health Care gives someone called a proxy the power to make health care decisions for the person with AD
- Living Will states the person's wishes for health care at the end of life
- Do Not Resuscitate (DNR) Form tells health care staff how the person wants end-of-life health care managed
- Will tells how the person wants his or her property and money to be divided among those left behind
- Living Trust tells someone called a trustee how to distribute a person's property and money

INFORMATION ON PLANNING

Contact the Alzheimer's Disease Education and Referral (ADEAR) Center at 1-800-438-4380 or www.nia.nih.gov/alzheimers for more information on planning for health, legal, and financial matters.

Check for money problems

People with AD often have problems managing their money. As the disease gets worse, a person may try to hide financial problems to protect his or her independence. Or, the person may not realize that he or she is losing the ability to handle money matters. Someone should check each month to see how the person is doing. This person might be a family member or the trustee.

Protect the person from fraud

People with AD also may be victims of financial abuse or "scams" by dishonest people. There can be telephone, mail, e-mail, or in-person scams. Sometimes, the person behind the scam is a "friend" or family member.

Scams can take many forms, such as:

- Identity theft
- Get-rich-quick offers
- Phony offers of prizes or home or auto repairs
- Insurance scams
- Threats

Here are some signs that the person with AD is not managing money well or has become a victim of a scam:

- The person seems afraid or worried when he or she talks about money.
- Money is missing from the person's bank account.
- Signatures on checks or other papers don't look like the person's signature.
- Bills are not being paid, and the person doesn't know why.
- The person's will has been changed without his or her permission.
- The person's home is sold, and he or she did not agree to sell it.

- Things that belong to you or the person with AD, such as clothes or jewelry, are missing from the home.
- The person has signed legal papers (such as a will, a power of attorney, or a joint deed to a house) without knowing what the papers mean.

Reporting Problems

If you think the person may be a victim of a scam, contact your local police department. You also can contact your state consumer protection office or Area Agency on Aging office. Look in the telephone book for a listing in the blue/Government pages or check the Internet.

Keeping the Person with AD Safe

Home safety

Over time, people with AD become less able to manage things around the house.

For example, they may forget:

- To turn off the oven or the water
- How to use the phone in an emergency
- Which things around the house, such as certain medicines or household cleaners, are dangerous
- Where things are in their own home

As a caregiver, you can do many things to make a house safer for people with AD.

Add the following to your home if you don't already have them in place:

- Smoke and carbon monoxide alarms in or near the kitchen and in all bedrooms
- Emergency phone numbers (ambulance, poison control, doctors, hospital, etc.) and your home address near all telephones
- Safety knobs on the stove and a shut-off switch

- Childproof plugs for unused electrical outlets

Lock up or remove the following from your home:

- All prescription and over-the-counter medicines
- Alcohol
- Cleaning products, dangerous chemicals such as paint thinner, matches, etc.
- Poisonous plants—contact the National Poison Control Center at 1-800-222-1222 or www.poison.org to find out which houseplants are poisonous
- All guns and other weapons, scissors, and knives
- Gasoline cans and other dangerous items in the garage

USE SIGNS

People with AD are able to read until the late stage of the disease. Use signs with simple written instructions to remind them of danger or show them where to go.

Do the following to keep the person with AD safe:

- Simplify your home. Too much furniture can make it hard to move freely.
- Get rid of clutter, such as piles of newspapers and magazines.
- Have a sturdy handrail on your stairway. Put carpet on stairs or add safety grip strips.
- Remove small throw rugs.
- Put a gate across the stairs if the person has balance problems.

- Make sure the person with AD has good floor traction for walking or pacing. Good traction lowers the chance that people will slip and fall. Three factors affect traction:

    1. The kind of floor surface. A smooth or waxed floor of tile, linoleum, or wood may be a problem for the person with AD. Think about how you might make the floor less slippery.
    2. Spills. Watch carefully for spills and clean them up right away.
    3. Shoes. Buy shoes and slippers with good traction. Look at the bottom of the shoe to check the type of material and tread.

Other home safety tips

People with AD get more confused over time. They also may not see, smell, touch, hear, and/or taste things as they used to.

You can do things around the house to make life safer and easier for the person with AD:

Seeing

- Make floors and walls different colors. This creates contrast and makes it easier for the person to see.
- Remove curtains and rugs with busy patterns that may confuse the person.
- Mark the edges of steps with brightly colored tape so people can see the steps as they go up or down stairs.
- Use brightly colored signs or simple pictures to label the bathroom, bedroom, and kitchen.
- Be careful about small pets. The person with AD may not see the pet and trip over it.
- Limit the size and number of mirrors in your home, and think about where to put them. Mirror images may confuse the person with AD.

Touching

- Reset your water heater to 120 degrees Fahrenheit to prevent burns.
- Label hot-water faucets red and cold-water faucets blue or write the words “hot” and “cold” near them.

- Put signs near the oven, toaster, iron, and other things that get hot. The sign could say, “Stop!” or “Don’t Touch—Very Hot!” Be sure the sign is not so close that it could catch on fire.
- Pad any sharp corners on your furniture, or replace or remove furniture with sharp corners.
- Test water in the bathtub by touching it, or use a thermometer to see whether it’s too hot. Water should not be above 120 degrees Fahrenheit.

Smelling

- Use good smoke detectors. People with AD may not be able to smell smoke.
- Check foods in your refrigerator often. Throw out any that have gone bad.

Tasting

- Keep foods like salt, sugar, and spices away from the person if you see him or her using too much.
- Put away or lock up things like toothpaste, lotions, shampoos, rubbing alcohol, soap, or perfume. They may look and smell like food to a person with AD.
- Keep the poison control number (1-800-222-1222) by the phone.
- Learn what to do if the person chokes on something. Check with your local Red Cross chapter about health or safety classes.

Hearing

- Don’t play the TV, CD player, or radio too loudly, and don’t play them at the same time. Loud music or too many different sounds may be too much for the person with AD to handle.
- Limit the number of people who visit at any one time. If there is a party, settle the person with AD in an area with fewer people.
- Shut the windows if it’s very noisy outside.
- If the person wears a hearing aid, check the batteries and settings often.

HOME SAFETY

To learn more about how to make your home a safe place inside and out, go to www.nia.nih.gov/alzheimers, and search for "home safety."

Driving safety

Good drivers are alert, think clearly, and make good decisions. When the person with AD is not able to do these things, he or she should stop driving. But, he or she may not want to stop or even think there is a problem. As the caregiver, you will need to talk with the person about why he or she needs to stop driving. Do this in a caring way. Understand how unhappy the person with AD may be that he or she has reached this new stage.

Be ready to find other ways that the person can travel on his or her own, for as long as possible. Your local Area Agency on Aging has information about transportation services in your area. These services may include free or low-cost buses, taxi service, or carpools for older people. Some churches and community groups have volunteers who take seniors wherever they want to go.

Here are some things you need to know about driving and memory loss:

- A person with some memory loss may be able to drive safely sometimes. But, he or she may not be able to react quickly when faced with a surprise on the road. This can be dangerous. If the person's reaction time slows, then you need to stop the person from driving.
- The person may be able to drive short distances on local streets during the day, but may not be able to drive safely at night or on a freeway. If this is the case, then limit the times and places that the person can drive.
- Some people with memory problems decide on their own not to drive. Others don't want to stop driving and may deny that they have a problem.

Here are some signs that the person should stop driving:

- New dents and scratches on the car
- Taking a long time to do a simple errand and not being able to explain why. That may indicate that the person got lost.

PLEASE REMEMBER

If the person with AD keeps driving when it is no longer safe, someone could get hurt or be killed. You need to weigh the danger to other people if he or she does drive against the feelings of the person. Talk to the person's doctor about this problem.

Also, consider asking a friend or family member to follow the person. What he or she sees can give you a better sense of how well the person with AD is driving.

Here are some ways to stop people with AD from driving:

- Try talking about your concerns with the person.
- Ask your doctor to tell him or her to stop driving. The doctor can write, "Do not drive" on a prescription pad and you can show this to the person. Some State Departments of Motor Vehicles require doctors to tell them if the person with AD should no longer drive.
- Ask family or friends to drive the person.
- Take him or her to get a driving test.
- Hide the car keys, move the car, take out the distributor cap, or disconnect the battery if the person won't stop driving.
- Find out about services that help people with disabilities get around their community. Look in the blue pages of your local telephone book, contact your local Area Agency on Aging office, or call the Community Transportation Association at 1-800-891-0590.
- If the person won't stop driving, contact your State Department of Motor Vehicles. Ask about a medical review for a person who may not be able to drive safely. He or she may be asked to retake a driving test. In some cases, the person's license could be taken away.

Providing Everyday Care for People with AD

Activity and exercise

Being active and getting exercise helps people with AD feel better. Exercise helps keep their muscles, joints, and heart in good shape. It also helps people stay at a healthy weight and have regular toilet and sleep habits. You can exercise together to make it more fun.

You want someone with AD to do as much as possible for himself or herself. At the same time, you also need to make sure that the person is safe when active.

Here are some tips for helping the person with AD stay active:

- Take a walk together each day. Exercise is good for caregivers, too!
- Make sure the person with AD has an ID bracelet with your phone number if he or she walks alone.
- Check your local TV guide to see if there is a program to help older adults exercise.
- Add music to the exercises if it helps the person with AD. Dance to the music if possible.
- Watch exercise videos/DVDs made for older people. Try exercising together.
- Make sure he or she wears comfortable clothes and shoes that fit well and are made for exercise.
- Make sure the person drinks water or juice after exercise.
- For more information on exercise and physical activity, visit www.nia.nih.gov/Go4Life or call 1-800-222-2225.

Some people with AD may not be able to get around well. This is another problem that becomes more challenging to deal with as the disease gets worse.

Some possible reasons for this include:

- Trouble with endurance
- Poor coordination
- Sore feet or muscles
- Illness
- Depression or general lack of interest

Even if people have trouble walking, they may be able to:

- Do simple tasks around the home, such as sweeping and dusting.
- Use a stationary bike.
- Use soft rubber exercise balls or balloons for stretching or throwing back and forth.
- Use stretching bands, which you can buy in sporting goods stores. Be sure to follow the instructions.

Healthy eating

Eating healthy foods helps us stay well. It’s even more important for people with AD. Here are some tips for healthy eating.

When the person with AD lives with you:

- Buy healthy foods such as vegetables, fruits, and whole-grain products. Be sure to buy foods that the person likes and can eat.
- Buy food that is easy to prepare, such as pre-made salads and single food portions.
- Have someone else make meals if possible.
- Use a service such as Meals on Wheels, which will bring meals right to your home. For more information, check your local phone book, or contact the Meals on Wheels organization at 1-888-998-6325 (www.mowaa.org).

When a person with early-stage AD lives alone:

- Follow the steps above.
- Buy foods that the person doesn’t need to cook.
- Call to remind him or her to eat.

In the early stage of AD, the person’s eating habits usually don’t change. When changes do occur, living alone may not be safe anymore.

Look for these signs to see if living alone is no longer safe for the person with AD:

- The person forgets to eat.

- Food has burned because it was left on the stove.
- The oven isn't turned off.

Everyday care

At some point, people with AD will need help bathing, combing their hair, brushing their teeth, and getting dressed. Because these are private activities, people may not want help. They may feel embarrassed about being naked in front of caregivers. They also may feel angry about not being able to care for themselves. Below are suggestions that may help with everyday care.

Bathing

Helping someone with AD take a bath or shower can be one of the hardest things you do. Planning can help make the person's bath time better for both of you.

The person with AD may be afraid. If so, follow the person's lifelong bathing habits, such as doing the bath or shower in the morning or before going to bed. Here are other tips for bathing.

Safety tips:

- Never leave a confused or frail person alone in the tub or shower.
- Always check the water temperature before he or she gets in the tub or shower.
- Use plastic containers for shampoo or soap to prevent them from breaking.
- Use a hand-held showerhead.
- Use a rubber bath mat and put safety bars in the tub.
- Use a sturdy shower chair in the tub or shower. This will support a person who is unsteady, and it could prevent falls. You can get shower chairs at drug stores and medical supply stores.

Before a bath or shower:

- Get the soap, washcloth, towels, and shampoo ready.
- Make sure the bathroom is warm and well lighted. Play soft music if it helps to relax the person.

- Be matter-of-fact about bathing. Say, "It's time for a bath now." Don't argue about the need for a bath or shower.
- Be gentle and respectful. Tell the person what you are going to do, step-by-step.
- Make sure the water temperature in the bath or shower is comfortable.
- Don't use bath oil. It can make the tub slippery and may cause urinary tract infections.

During a bath or shower:

- Allow the person with AD to do as much as possible. This protects his or her dignity and helps the person feel more in control.
- Put a towel over the person's shoulders or lap. This helps him or her feel less exposed. Then use a sponge or washcloth to clean under the towel.
- Distract the person by talking about something else if he or she becomes upset.
- Give him or her a washcloth to hold. This makes it less likely that the person will try to hit you.

After a bath or shower:

- Prevent rashes or infections by patting the person's skin with a towel. Make sure the person is completely dry. Be sure to dry between folds of skin.
- If the person has trouble with incontinence, use a protective ointment, such as Vaseline®, around the rectum, vagina, or penis.
- If the person with AD has trouble getting in and out of the bathtub, do a sponge bath instead.

Other bathing tips:

- Give the person a full bath two or three times a week. For most people, a sponge bath to clean the face, hands, feet, underarms, and genital or "private" area is all you need to do every day.
- Washing the person's hair in the sink may be easier than doing it in the shower or bathtub. You can buy a hose attachment for the sink.

- Get professional help with bathing if it becomes too hard for you to do on your own.

Grooming

For the most part, when people feel good about how they look, they feel better. Helping people with AD brush their teeth, shave, or put on makeup often means they can feel more like themselves. Here are some grooming tips.

Mouth care:

Good mouth care helps prevent dental problems such as cavities and gum disease.

- Show the person how to brush his or her teeth. Go step-by-step. For example, pick up the toothpaste, take the top off, put the toothpaste on the toothbrush, and then brush. Remember to let the person do as much as possible.
- Brush your teeth at the same time.
- Help the person clean his or her dentures. Make sure he or she uses the denture cleaning material the right way.
- Ask the person to rinse his or her mouth with water after each meal and use mouthwash once a day.
- Try a long-handled, angled, or electric toothbrush if you need to brush the person's teeth.
- Take the person to see a dentist. Some dentists specialize in treating people with AD. Be sure to follow the dentist's advice about how often to make an appointment.

Other grooming tips:

- Encourage a woman to wear makeup if she has always used it. If needed, help her put on powder and lipstick. Don't use eye makeup.
- Encourage a man to shave, and help him as needed. Use an electric razor for safety.
- Take the person to the barber or beauty shop. Some barbers or hairstylists may come to your home.
- Keep the person's nails clean and trimmed.

Dressing

People with AD often need more time to dress. It can be hard for them to choose their clothes. They might wear the wrong clothing for the season. They also might wear colors that don't go together or forget to put on a piece of clothing. Allow the person to dress on his or her own for as long as possible.

Other tips include the following:

- Lay out clothes in the order the person should put them on, such as underwear first, then pants, then a shirt, and then a sweater.
- Hand the person one thing at a time or give step-by-step dressing instructions.
- Put away some clothes in another room to reduce the number of choices. Keep only one or two outfits in the closet or dresser.
- Keep the closet locked if needed. This prevents some of the problems people may have while getting dressed.
- Buy three or four sets of the same clothes, if the person wants to wear the same clothing every day.
- Buy loose-fitting, comfortable clothing. Avoid girdles, control-top pantyhose, knee-high nylons, garters, high heels, tight socks, and bras for women. Sports bras are comfortable and provide good support. Short cotton socks and loose cotton underwear are best. Sweat pants and shorts with elastic waistbands are helpful.
- Use Velcro® tape or large zipper pulls for clothing, instead of shoelaces, buttons, or buckles. Try slip-on shoes that won't slide off or shoes with Velcro® straps.

Adapting Activities for People with AD

Doing things we enjoy gives us pleasure and adds meaning to our lives. People with AD need to be active and do things they enjoy. However, don't expect too much. It's not easy for them to plan their days and do different tasks.

Here are two reasons:

- They may have trouble deciding what to do each day. This could make them fearful and worried or quiet and withdrawn.

- They may have trouble starting tasks. Remember, the person is not being lazy. He or she might need help organizing the day or doing an activity.

Daily activities

Plan activities that the person with AD enjoys. He or she can be a part of the activity or just watch. Also, you don't always have to be the "activities director."

Here are things you can do to help the person enjoy an activity:

- Match the activity with what the person with AD can do.
- Choose activities that can be fun for everyone.
- Help the person get started.
- Decide if he or she can do the activity alone or needs help.
- Watch to see if the person gets frustrated.
- Make sure he or she feels successful and has fun.
- Let him or her watch if that is more enjoyable.

The person with AD can do different activities each day. This keeps the day interesting and fun. The following pages may give you some ideas.

Household chores

Doing household chores can boost the person's self-esteem. When the person helps you, don't forget to say "thank you."

The person could:

- Wash dishes, set the table, or prepare food.
- Sweep the floor.
- Polish shoes.
- Sort mail and clip coupons.
- Sort socks and fold laundry.
- Sort recycling materials or other things.

Cooking and baking

Cooking and baking can bring the person with AD a lot of joy.

He or she might help do the following:

- Decide on what is needed to prepare the dish.
- Make the dish.
- Measure, mix, and pour.
- Tell someone else how to prepare a recipe.
- Taste the food.
- Watch others prepare food.

Children

Being around children also can be fun. It gives the person with AD someone to talk with and may bring back happy memories. It also can help the person realize how much he or she still can love others and can still be loved.

Here are some things the person might enjoy doing with children:

- Play a simple board game.
- Read stories or books.
- Visit family members who have small children.
- Walk in the park or around schoolyards.
- Go to sports or school events that involve young people.
- Talk about fond memories from childhood.

Music and dancing

Music can bring back happy memories and feelings. Some people feel the rhythm and may want to dance. Others enjoy listening to or talking about their favorite music. Even if the person with AD has trouble finding the right words to speak, he or she still may be able to sing songs from the past.

Consider the following musical activities:

- Play CDs, tapes, or records.
- Talk about the music and the singer.
- Ask what he or she was doing when the song was popular.
- Talk about the music and past events.
- Sing or dance to well-known songs.
- Play musical games like “Name That Tune.”
- Attend a concert or musical program.

Pets

Many people with AD enjoy pets, such as dogs, cats, or birds. Pets may help "bring them to life." Pets also can help people feel more loved and less worried.

Suggested activities with pets include:

- Care for, feed, or groom the pet.
- Walk the pet.
- Sit and hold the pet.

Gardening

Gardening is a way to be part of nature. It also may help people remember past days and fun times. Gardening can help the person focus on what he or she still can do.

Here are some suggested gardening activities:

- Take care of indoor or outdoor plants.
- Plant flowers and vegetables.
- Water the plants when needed.
- Talk about how much the plants are growing.

Going out

Early in the disease, people with AD may still enjoy the same kinds of outings they enjoyed in the past. Keep going on these outings as long as you are comfortable doing them.

Plan outings for the time of day when the person is at his or her best. Keep outings from becoming too long. You want to note how tired the person with AD gets after a certain amount of time (1/2 hour, 1 hour, 2 hours, etc.).

The person might enjoy outings to a:

- Favorite restaurant
- Zoo, park, or shopping mall
- Swimming pool (during a slow time of day at the pool)
- Museum, theater, or art exhibits for short trips

Remember that you can use a business-size card, as shown below, to tell others about the person's disease. Sharing the information with store clerks or restaurant staff can make outings more comfortable for everyone.

> My family member has Alzheimer's disease. He might say or do things that are unexpected. Thank you for your understanding.

Eating out

Going out to eat can be a welcome change. But, it also can have some challenges. Planning can help. You need to think about the layout of the restaurant, the menu, the noise level, waiting times, and the helpfulness of staff. Below are some tips for eating out with the person who has AD.

Before choosing a restaurant, ask yourself:

- Does the person with AD know the restaurant well?
- Is it quiet or noisy most of time?
- Are tables easy to get to? Do you need to wait before you can be seated?
- Is the service quick enough to keep the person from getting restless?
- Does the restroom meet the person's needs?
- Are foods the person with AD likes on the menu?
- Is the staff understanding and helpful?

Before going to the restaurant, decide:

- If it is a good day to go.
- When is the best time to go. Going out earlier in the day may be best, so the person is not too tired. Service may be quicker, and there may be fewer people. If you decide to go later, try to get the person to take a nap first.
- What you will take with you. You may need to take utensils, a towel, wipes, or toilet items that the person already uses. If so, make sure this is OK with the restaurant.

At the restaurant:

- Tell the waiter or waitress about any special needs, such as extra spoons, bowls, or napkins.
- Ask for a table near the washroom and in a quiet area.
- Seat the person with his or her back to the busy areas.
- Help the person choose his or her meal, if needed. Suggest food you know the person likes. Read parts of the menu or show the person a picture of the food. Limit the number of choices.
- Ask the waiter or waitress to fill glasses half full or leave the drinks for you to serve.
- Order some finger food or snacks to hold the attention of the person with AD.
- Go with the person to the restroom. Go into the stall if the person needs help.

Traveling

Taking the person with AD on a trip is a challenge. Traveling can make the person more worried and confused. Planning can make travel easier for everyone. Below are some tips that you may find helpful.

Before you leave on the trip:

- Talk with your doctor about medicines to calm someone who gets upset while traveling.
- Find someone to help you at the airport or train station.
- Keep important documents with you in a safe place. These include: insurance cards, passports, doctor's name and phone number, list of medicines, and a copy of medical records.
- Pack items the person enjoys looking at or holding for comfort.
- Travel with another family member or friend.
- Take an extra set of clothing in a carry-on bag.

After you arrive:

- Allow lots of time for each thing you want to do. Do not plan too many activities.
- Plan rest periods.

- Follow a routine like the one you use at home. For example, try to have the person eat, rest, and go to bed at the same time he or she does at home.
- Keep a well-lighted path to the toilet, and leave the bathroom light on all night.
- Be prepared to cut your visit short.

People with memory problems may wander around a place they don't know well.

In case someone with AD gets lost:

- Make sure they wear or have something with them that tells who they are, such as an ID bracelet.
- Carry a recent photo of the person with you on the trip.

Spiritual activities

Like you, the person with AD may have spiritual needs. If so, you can help the person stay part of his or her faith community. This can help the person feel connected to others and remember pleasant times.

Here are some tips for helping a person with AD who has spiritual needs:

- Involve the person in spiritual activities that he or she has known well. These might include worship, religious or other readings, sacred music, prayer, and holiday rituals.
- Tell people in your faith community that the person has AD. Encourage them to talk with the person and show him or her that they still care.
- Play religious or other music that is important to the person. It may bring back old memories. Even if the person with AD has a problem finding the right words to speak, he or she still may be able to sing songs or hymns from the past.

Holidays

Many caregivers have mixed feelings about holidays. They may have happy memories of the past. But, they also may worry about the extra demands that holidays make on their time and energy.

Here are some suggestions to help you find a balance between doing many holiday-related things and resting:

- Celebrate holidays that are important to you. Include the person with AD as much as possible.
- Understand that things will be different. Be realistic about what you can do.
- Ask friends and family to visit. Limit the number of visitors at any one time. Plan visits when the person usually is at his or her best (see the section about "Visitors").
- Avoid crowds, changes in routine, and strange places that may make the person with AD feel confused or nervous.
- Do your best to enjoy yourself. Find time for the holiday activities you like to do. Ask a friend or family member to spend time with the person while you're out.
- Make sure there is a space where the person can rest when he or she goes to larger gatherings such as weddings or family reunions.

Visitors

Visitors are important to people with AD. They may not always remember who visitors are, but they often enjoy the company.

Here are ideas to share with a person planning to visit someone with AD:

- Plan the visit when the person with AD is at his or her best.
- Consider bringing along some kind of activity, such as a well-known book or photo album to look at. This can help if the person is bored or confused and needs to be distracted. But, be prepared to skip the activity if it is not needed.
- Be calm and quiet. Don't use a loud voice or talk to the person as if he or she were a child.
- Respect the person's personal space, and don't get too close.
- Make eye contact and call the person by name to get his or her attention.
- Remind the person who you are if he or she doesn't seem to know you.

- Don't argue if the person is confused. Respond to the feelings that they express. Try to distract the person by talking about something different.
- Remember not to take it personally if the person doesn't recognize you, is unkind, or gets angry. He or she is acting out of confusion.

WHEN YOU NEED HELP

Getting Help with Caregiving

Some caregivers need help when the person is in the early stages of AD. Other caregivers look for help when the person is in the later stages of AD. It's okay to seek help whenever you need it.

As the person moves through the stages of AD, he or she will need more care. One reason is that medicines used to treat AD can only control symptoms; they cannot cure the disease. Symptoms, such as memory loss and confusion, will get worse over time. Because of this, you will need more help. You may feel that asking for help shows weakness or a lack of caring, but the opposite is true. Asking for help shows your strength. It means you know your limits and when to seek support.

Build a support system

According to many caregivers, building a local support system is a key way to get help. Your support system might include your caregiver support group, the local chapter of the Alzheimer's Association, family, friends, and faith groups. Call the ADEAR Center at 1-800-438-4380, the Alzheimer's Association at 1-800-272-3900, and the Eldercare Locator at 1-800-677-1116 to learn about where to get help in your community. On the following pages, we list other national and local resources that can help you with caregiving.

Information resources

Here are some places along with their phone numbers that can give you support and advice:

Alzheimer's Disease Education and Referral (ADEAR) Center
P.O. Box 8250 Silver Spring, MD 20907-8250
Phone: 1-800-438-4380
www.nia.nih.gov/alzheimers

The ADEAR Center offers information on diagnosis, treatment, patient care, caregiver needs, long-term care, and research and clinical trials related to AD. Staff can refer you to local and national resources, or you can search for information on the website. The Center is a service of the National Institute on Aging, part of the Federal Government's National Institutes of Health. They have information to help you understand Alzheimer's disease. You can also get hints on other subjects, including:

- talking with the doctor
- financial and legal planning
- medicines
- comfort care at the end of life

Alzheimer's Association
225 N. Michigan Avenue
Floor 17
Chicago, IL 60601
Phone: 1-800-272-3900
www.alz.org

The Alzheimer's Association offers information, a help line, and support services to people with AD and their caregivers. Local chapters across the country offer support groups, including many that help with early-stage AD. Call or go online to find out where to get help in your area. The Association also funds AD research.

Alzheimer's Foundation of America
322 Eighth Avenue, 7th Floor
New York, NY 10001
Phone: 1-866-232-8484
www.alzfdn.org

The Alzheimer's Foundation of America provides information about how to care for people with AD as well as a list of services for people with AD. It also offers information for caregivers and their families through member organizations. Services include a toll-free hotline, publications, and other educational materials.

Eldercare Locator
Phone: 1-800-677-1116
www.eldercare.gov

Caregivers often need information about community resources, such as home care, adult day care, and nursing homes. Contact the Eldercare Locator to find these resources in your area. The Eldercare Locator is a service of the Administration on Aging. The Federal Government funds this service.

National Institute on Aging Information Center
P.O. Box 8057
Gaithersburg, MD 20898-8057
Phone: 1-800-222-2225
TTY: 1-800-222-4225
www.nia.nih.gov/health

The NIA Information Center offers free helpful publications about aging. Many of these publications are in both English and Spanish. They can be viewed, printed, and ordered from the Internet. The NIA, along with the National Library of Medicine, also offers a website specially designed for seniors called NIHSeniorHealth, which is available at www.nihseniorhealth.gov.

Direct services—groups that help with everyday care in the home

Here is a list of services that can help you care for the person with AD at home. Find out if these services are offered in your area. Also, contact Medicare to see if they cover the cost of any of these services.

Home Health Care Services

What they do:

Send a home health aide to your home to help you care for a person with AD. These aides provide care and/or company for the person. They may come for a few hours or stay for 24 hours. Some home health aides are better trained and supervised than others.

What to know about costs:

- Home health services charge by the hour.
- Medicare covers some home health service costs.
- Most insurance plans do not cover these costs.
- You must pay all costs not covered by Medicare, Medicaid, or insurance.

How to find them:

- Ask your doctor or other health care professional about good home health care services in your area.
- Look in your phone book under "home health care."

HOME HEALTH CARE SERVICES

Some home health care services are very good; others are not. You should get as much information as possible about a service before you sign an agreement. You need to ask home health care providers for references from people who have used their services. If possible, check for any complaints filed against a service. At Medicare's Home Health Compare, www.medicare.gov/HomeHealthCompare, you can learn more about some of the home health care providers in your state. Or call Medicare for the same information. You can also check with community, county, or State agencies that regulate health services or contact the Better Business Bureau in your area.

Here are some questions you might ask before signing a home health care agreement:

- Is your service licensed and accredited?
- What is the cost of your services?
- What is included and not included in your services?
- How many days a week and hours a day will an aide come to my home?
- How do you check the background and experience of your home health aides?
- How do you train your home health aides?

- Can I get special help in an emergency?
- What types of emergency care can you provide?
- Whom do I contact if there is a problem?

Meal services

What they do:

- Bring hot meals to the person's home or your home. The delivery staff do not feed the person.

What to know about costs:

- The person with AD must qualify for the service based on local guidelines.
- Some groups do not charge for their services. Others may charge a small fee.

How to find them:

- The Eldercare Locator can help at 1-800-677-1116 or www.eldercare.gov. Or, call the Meals on Wheels organization at 1-888-998-6325 or visit their website at www.mowaa.org.

Adult day care services

What they do:

- Provide a safe environment, activities, and staff who pay attention to the needs of the person with AD in an adult day care facility
- Provide a much-needed break for you
- Provide transportation—the facility may pick up the person, take him or her to day care, and then return the person home

What to know about costs:

- Adult day care services charge by the hour.

- Most insurance plans don't cover these costs. You must pay all costs not covered by insurance.

How to find them:

- Call the National Adult Day Services Association at 1-877-745-1440, or visit their website at www.nadsa.org. You also can call the Eldercare Locator at 1-800-677-1116, or visit their website at www.eldercare.gov.

Respite services

What they do:

- Provide short stays, from a few days to a few weeks, in a nursing home or other place for the person with AD
- Allow you to get a break to rest or go on a vacation

What to know about costs:

- Respite services charge by the number of days or weeks that services are provided.
- Medicare or Medicaid may cover the cost of up to 5 days in a row of respite care in an inpatient facility.
- Most insurance plans do not cover these costs.
- You must pay all costs not covered by Medicare, Medicaid, or insurance.

How to find them:

- Visit the National Respite Locator Service at www.respitelocator.org.

Geriatric care managers

What they do:

- Make a home visit and suggest needed services
- Help you get needed services

What to know about costs:

- Geriatric care managers charge by the hour.
- Most insurance plans don't cover these costs.
- Medicare does not pay for this service.
- You will probably have to pay for this service.

How to find them:

- Call the National Association of Professional Geriatric Care Managers at 1-520-881-8008, or visit its website at www.caremanager.org.

Counseling from a mental health or social work professional

What they do:

- Help you deal with any stress you may be feeling
- Help you understand your feelings, such as anger, sadness, or feeling out of control and overwhelmed
- Help develop plans for unexpected or sudden events

What to know about costs:

- Professional mental health counselors charge by the hour. There may be big differences in the rates you would be charged from one counselor to another.
- Some insurance companies will cover some of these costs.
- Medicare or Medicaid may cover some of these costs.
- You must pay all costs not covered by Medicare, Medicaid, or insurance.

How to find them:

- It's a good idea to ask your health insurance staff which counselors and services, if any, your insurance plan covers. Then check with your doctor, local family service agencies, and community mental health agencies for referrals to counselors.

Hospice services

What they do:

- Provide care for a person who is near the end of life
- Keep the person who is dying as comfortable and pain-free as possible
- Provide care in the home or in a hospice facility
- Support the family in providing in-home or end-of-life care

What to know about costs:

- Hospice services charge by the number of days or weeks that services are provided.
- Medicare or Medicaid may cover hospice costs.
- Most insurance plans do not cover these costs.
- You must pay all costs not covered by Medicare, Medicaid, or insurance.

How to find them:

- American Hospice Foundation at 1-202-223-0204 or www.americanhospice.org
- National Association for Home Care and Hospice at 1-202-547-7424 or www.nahc.org
- Hospice Foundation of America at 1-800-854-3402 or www.hospicefoundation.org
- National Hospice and Palliative Care Organization at 1-800-658-8898 or www.caringinfo.org

Government benefits—financial help from Federal and State Government programs

Federal and State Government programs can provide financial support and services.

Medicare

Medicare is a Federal Government health insurance program that pays some medical costs for people age 65 and older. It also pays some medical costs for those who have gotten Social Security Disability Income (discussed later in this section) for 24 months.

Here are brief descriptions of what Medicare will pay for:

Medicare Part A

- Hospital costs after you pay a certain amount, called the “deductible”
- Short stays in a nursing home for certain kinds of illnesses

Medicare Part B

- 80 percent of the costs for certain services, such as doctor’s fees, some tests, x-rays, and medical equipment

Medicare Part D

- Some medication costs

You can find more information about Medicare benefits on the Internet at www.medicare.gov, or call 1-800-633-4227, TTY: 1-877-486-2048.

Medicaid

Medicaid is a combined Federal and State program for low-income people and families. Medicaid will pay the costs of some types of long-term care for some people and their families. You must meet certain financial requirements.

To learn more about Medicaid:
Phone: 1-877-267-2323
TTY: 1-866-226-1819
www.medicaid.gov

Or, contact your state health department. For a state-by-state list, visit www.medicaid.gov/Medicaid-CHIP-Program-Information/By-State/By-State.html.

Program of All-Inclusive Care for the Elderly (PACE)

PACE is a program that combines Medicare and Medicaid benefits. PACE may pay for some or all of the long-term care needs of the person with AD. It covers medical, social service, and long-term care costs for frail people. PACE permits most people who qualify to continue living at home instead of moving to a long-term care facility. PACE is available only in certain States and locations within those States. Also, there may be a monthly charge. You will need to find out if the person qualifies for PACE.

To find out more about PACE:
Phone: 1-800-772-1213
www.medicare.gov/nursing/alternatives/pace.asp

Social Security Disability Income

This type of Social Security help is for people younger than age 65 who are disabled according to the Social Security Administration's definition.

You must be able to show that:

- The person with AD is unable to work, and
- The condition will last at least a year, or
- The condition is expected to result in death.

Social Security has "compassionate allowances" to help people with early-onset Alzheimer's disease, mixed dementia, frontotemporal dementia/Pick's disease, primary progressive aphasia, and certain other serious medical conditions get disability benefits more quickly.

To find out more about Social Security Disability Income:
Phone: 1-800-772-1213
TTY: 1-800-325-0778
www.socialsecurity.gov

State Health Insurance Assistance Program (SHIP)

SHIP is a national program offered in each State that provides free counseling and advice about coverage and benefits to people with Medicare and their families. To contact a SHIP counselor in your State, visit www.shiptalk.org.

Department of Veterans Affairs

The U.S. Department of Veterans Affairs (VA) may provide long-term care for some veterans. There could be a waiting list for VA nursing homes. The VA also provides some at-home care.

To learn more about VA healthcare benefits:
Phone: 1-877-222-8387
www.va.gov/health

National Council on Aging

The National Council on Aging, a private group, has a free service called BenefitsCheckUp. This service can help you find Federal and State benefit programs that may help your family. These programs can help pay for prescription drugs, heating bills, housing, meal programs, and legal services.

BenefitsCheckUp also can help you find:

- Financial assistance
- Veteran's benefits
- Employment/volunteer work
- Helpful information and resources

To learn more about BenefitsCheckUp:
Phone: 1-202-479-1200
www.benefitscheckup.org

Finding the Right Place for the Person with AD

Sometimes you can no longer care for the person with AD at home. The person may need around-the-clock care. Or, he or she may be incontinent, aggressive, or wander a lot. It may not be possible for you to meet all of his or her needs at home anymore. When that happens, you may want to look for another place for the person with AD to live. You may feel guilty or upset about this decision, but remember that many caregivers reach this point as the disease worsens. Moving the person to a care facility may give you greater peace of mind. You will know that the person with AD is safe and getting good care.

Choosing the right place is a big decision. It's hard to know where to start.

Below we list steps you can take to find the right place:

1. **Gather information**

- Talk with your support group members, social worker, doctor, family members, and friends about facilities in your area.
- Make a list of questions to ask about the facility.
- Call to set up a time to visit.

Check these resources:

Centers for Medicare and Medicaid Services (CMS)
7500 Security Boulevard
Baltimore, MD 21244-1850
1-800-MEDICARE (1-800-633-4227)
TTY: 1-877-486-2048
www.medicare.gov

CMS has a guide to help older people and their caregivers choose a good nursing home. It describes types of long-term care, questions to ask the nursing home staff, and ways to pay for nursing home care. CMS also offers a service called Nursing Home Compare on its website. This service has information on nursing homes that are Medicare or Medicaid certified. These nursing homes provide skilled nursing care. Please note that there are many other places that provide different levels of health care and help with daily living. Many of these facilities are licensed only at the State level. CMS also has information about the rights of nursing home residents and their caregivers.

Joint Commission
One Renaissance Boulevard
Oakbrook Terrace, IL 60181
1-630-792-5800
www.qualitycheck.org
www.jointcommission.org

The Joint Commission evaluates nursing homes, home health care providers, hospitals, and assisted living facilities to determine whether or not they meet professional standards of care. Consumers can learn more about the quality of health care facilities through their online service at www.qualitycheck.org.

Other resources include:

AARP
601 E Street, NW
Washington, DC 20049
1-888-OUR-AARP (1-888-687-2277)
www.aarp.org/family/housing

Assisted Living Federation of America
1650 King Street, Suite 602
Alexandria, VA 22314
1-703-894-1805
www.alfa.org

National Center for Assisted Living
1201 L Street, NW
Washington, DC 20005
1-202-842-4444
www.ncal.org

National Clearinghouse for Long Term Care Information
Administration for Community Living
Washington, DC 20201
1-202-619-0724
www.longtermcare.gov

2. Visit assisted living facilities and nursing homes

Make several visits at different times of the day and evening.

Ask yourself:

- How does the staff care for the residents?
- Is the staff friendly?
- Does the place feel comfortable?
- How do the people who live there look?
- Do they look clean and well cared for?
- Are mealtimes comfortable?

- Is the facility clean and well maintained?
- Does it smell bad?

Ask the staff:

- What activities are planned for residents?
- How many staff members are at the facility? How many of them are trained to provide medical care if needed?
- How many people in the facility have AD?
- Does the facility have a special unit for people with AD? If so, what kinds of services does it provide?
- Is there a doctor who checks on residents on a regular basis? How often?

You also may want to ask staff:

- What is a typical day like for the person with AD?
- Is there a safe place for the person to go outside?
- How do staff members speak to residents—with respect?
- What is included in the fee?
- How does my loved one get to medical appointments?

Talk with other caregivers who have a loved one at the facility. Find out what they think about the place.

Find out about total costs of care. Each facility is different. You want to find out if long-term care insurance, Medicaid, or Medicare will pay for any of the costs. Remember that Medicare only covers nursing home costs for a short time after the person with AD has been in the hospital for a certain amount of time.

If you're asked to sign a contract, make sure you understand what you are agreeing to.

Assisted living facilities

Assisted living facilities have rooms or apartments. They're for people who can mostly take care of themselves, but may need some help. Some assisted living facilities have special AD units. These units have staff who check on and care for people with AD. You will need to pay for the cost of the room or apartment, and you may need to pay extra for any special care. Some assisted living facilities are part of a larger organization that also offers other levels of care. For example, continuing care retirement communities also offer independent living and skilled nursing care.

Group homes

A group home is a home for people who can no longer take care of themselves. Four to 10 people who can't care for themselves and two or more staff members live in the home. The staff takes care of the people living there: making meals, helping with grooming and medication, and providing other care. You will need to pay the costs of the person with AD living in this kind of home. Remember that these homes may not be inspected or regulated, but may still provide good care.

Check out the home and the staff. Visit at different times of the day and evening to see how the staff takes care of the residents. Also check to see how clean and comfortable the home is. You'll want to look at how the residents get along with one another and with the staff.

Nursing homes

Nursing homes are for people who can't care for themselves anymore. Some nursing homes have special AD care units. These units are often in separate sections of the building where staff members have special training to care for people with AD. Some units try to make the person feel more like he or she is at home. They provide special activities, meals, and medical care. In most cases, you will have to pay for nursing home care. Some nursing homes accept Medicaid as payment. Also, long-term care insurance may cover some of the nursing home costs. Nursing homes are inspected and regulated by State governments.

How to make moving day easier

Moving is very stressful. Moving the person with AD to an assisted living facility, group home, or nursing home is a big change for both the person and the caregiver. You may feel many emotions, from a sense of loss to guilt and sadness. You also may feel relieved. It is okay to have all these feelings. A social worker may be able to help you plan for and adjust to moving day. It's important to have support during this difficult step.

Here are some things that may help:

- Know that the day can be very stressful.
- Talk to a social worker about your feelings about moving the person into a new place. Find out how to help the person with AD adjust.
- Get to know the staff before the person moves into a facility.
- Talk with the staff about ways to make the change to the assisted living facility or nursing home go better.
- Don't argue with the person with AD about why he or she needs to be there.

Be an advocate

Once the person has moved to his or her new home, check and see how the person is doing. As the caregiver, you probably know the person best. Look for signs that the person may need more attention, is taking too much medication, or may not be getting the care they need. Build a relationship with staff so that you work together as partners.

The Medical Side of AD

Medicines to Treat AD Symptoms and Behaviors

This section contains medical terms and drug names.

People with AD may take medications to treat:

- The disease itself
- Mood or other behavior changes
- Other medical conditions they may have

Caregivers need to know about **each** medicine that a person with AD takes.

Ask the doctor or pharmacist the questions below and write down the answers:

- Why is this medicine being used?

- What positive effects should I look for, and when?
- How long will the person need to take it?
- How much should he or she take each day?
- When does the person need to take the medicine?
- What are the side effects?
- What can I do about these side effects?
- Can the medicine be crushed and mixed into foods such as applesauce?
- Can I get the medicine in a liquid form?
- Can this medicine cause problems if taken with other medicines?

Reminders to take medicine

People with AD often need help taking their medicine. If the person still lives alone, you may need to call and remind him or her. It's also helpful to buy a pillbox and put pills for each day in the box. That way all the pills for the day are in one place. You can get pillboxes at the drugstore. As the disease gets worse, you will need to keep track of his or her medicines. You also will need to make sure they take the medicine or you will need to give them the medicine. Ask the doctor or pharmacist about when to give the medications.

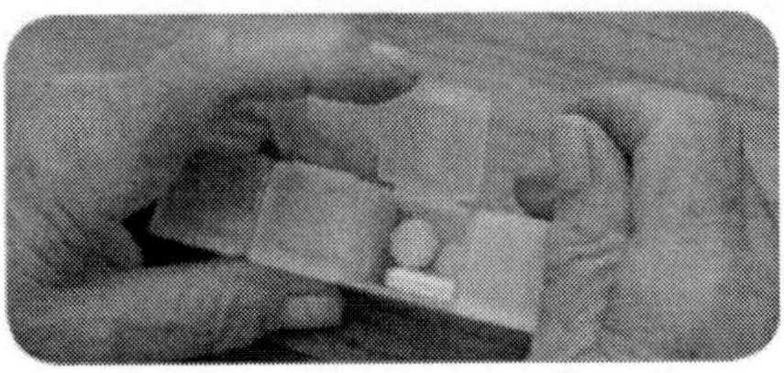

Medicines to treat AD

Both caregivers and doctors need to remember that no two people with AD are alike. This means that medications may work differently in different people.

Many factors may play a role in the disease, such as:

- Genes
- Lifestyle
- Earlier treatments
- Other illnesses or problems

- The person's surroundings
- Stage of AD

Work closely with the doctor to learn which medicines to use for AD, how much to use, and when to use them. Check with the doctor to see if Medicare or private insurance will cover the cost of the medicines. Also, find out if you can buy the non-brand, also called generic, type of the medicine. They often cost less than the brand name medicines.

When this chapter was written, four medicines were approved to treat AD. Other promising new medicines are being tested.

It's important to understand that none of the four medicines can cure or stop the disease. What they can do, for some people, is help them improve for a while from where they started. However, most of the time, these medicines work to slow down certain problems, such as memory loss. Slowing down memory loss can allow many people with AD to be more comfortable and independent for a longer time.

Medicines for mild to moderate AD

Three of the four medicines to treat AD are similar. They are used to treat mild to moderate stages of the disease. They may help delay or slow down some symptoms. One of the medicines, Aricept®, also may help people with severe AD.

The names of these three medicines are:

- Aricept® (AIR-uh-sept), brand name; donepezil (doe-NEP-uh-zil), generic name
- Exelon® (EKS-uh-lawn), brand name; rivastigmine (riv-uh-STIG-meen), generic name
- Razadyne® (RAZZ-uh-dine), brand name; galantamine (guh-LAN-tuh-meen), generic name

ASK THE DOCTOR ABOUT SIDE EFFECTS

Check with the doctor or pharmacist about any possible side effects of medication. Some side effects can be serious.

A medicine for moderate to severe AD

Namenda®, the fourth medicine, is used to treat moderate to severe AD. For some patients, Namenda® (nuh-MEN-duh) may delay or slow the symptoms of AD. This may allow some people to do more things for themselves, such as using the toilet. The generic name of this drug is memantine (MEH-man-teen).

Sometimes doctors use a combination of medicines to treat moderate to severe AD. For example, they might use Aricept® and Namenda®. These two medicines work in different ways, so it is safe to take them together.

Medicines to treat behavior problems related to AD

Examples of behavior problems that can occur in AD are restlessness, anxiety, depression, trouble sleeping, and aggression. Experts agree that medicines to treat these behavior problems should be used only after other strategies that don't use medicine have been tried. If they don't work and the person with AD continues to be upset, restless, depressed, or aggressive, he or she may need medicine. Talk with the doctor about which medicines are safest and most effective to help with these problems.

Remember the following tips about medicines:

- Use the lowest dose possible.
- Watch for side effects. Be prepared to stop the medicine if they occur.
- Allow the medicine a few weeks to take effect.

Below is a list of medicines used to help with depression, aggression, restlessness, and anxiety.

Antidepressants are drugs used to treat depression and worry (also called anxiety).

Examples of these medicines include:

- Celexa® (Sa-LEKS-a), brand name; citalopram (SYE-tal-oh-pram), generic name
- Remeron® (REM-er-on), brand name; mirtazepine (MUR-taz-a-peen), generic name
- Zoloft® (ZO-loft), brand name; sertraline (SUR-truh-leen), generic name

Know about Medicines

Information about medicines changes over time. Check with the doctor, AD specialist, or pharmacist about the latest medicines. The doctor may prescribe newer drugs with different names than those listed in this chapter. Also, remember that some medicines have both generic and brand names.

Anticonvulsants are drugs sometimes used to treat severe aggression.

Examples of these medicines include:

- Depakote® (DEP-uh-cote), brand name; sodium valproate (so-DEE-um VAL-pro-ate), generic name
- Tegretol® (TEG-ruh-tall), brand name; carbamazepine (KAR-ba-maz-ee-peen), generic name
- Trileptal® (tri-LEP-tall), brand name; oxcarbazepine (oks-kar-BAZ-eh-peen), generic name

Medicines to be used with caution

There are some medicines, such as sleep aids, anti-anxiety drugs, and antipsychotics, that the person with AD should take only:

- After the doctor has explained all the risks and side effects of the medicine
- After other, safer medicines have not helped treat the problem

You will need to watch closely for side effects from these medications.

Sleep aids are used to help people get to sleep and stay asleep. People with AD should NOT use these drugs on a regular basis because they make the person more confused and more likely to fall.

Examples of these medicines include:

- Ambien® (AM-bee-un), brand name; zolpidem (zole-PI-dem), generic name

- Lunesta® (lu-NES-ta), brand name; eszopiclone (ess-ZOP-eh-klone), generic name
- Sonata® (SO-nah-ta), brand name; zaleplon (ZAL-ee-plon), generic name

Anti-anxiety drugs are used to treat agitation. These drugs can cause sleepiness, dizziness, falls, and confusion. Therefore, doctors recommend using them only for short periods of time.

Examples of these medicines include:

- Ativan® (AT-eh-van), brand name; lorazepam (lor-AZ-eh-pam), generic name
- Klonopin® (KLON-uh-pin), brand name; clonazepam (klo-NAY-zeh-pam), generic name

Antipsychotics are drugs used to treat paranoia, hallucinations, agitation, and aggression. Side effects of using these drugs can be serious, including increased risk of death in some older people with dementia. They should ONLY be given to people with AD when the doctor agrees that the symptoms are severe.

Examples of these medicines include:

- Risperdal® (RISS-per-doll), brand name; risperidone (riss-PAIR-eh-dohn), generic name
- Seroquel® (SAIR-o-kwell), brand name; quetiapine (KWE-tye-uh-peen), generic name
- Zyprexa® (zye-PREKS-uh), brand name; olanzapine (o-LAN-zuh-peen), generic name

Medicines that people with AD should not take

Anticholinergic drugs are used to treat many medical problems such as sleeping problems, stomach cramps, incontinence, asthma, motion sickness, and muscle spasms. Side effects, such as confusion, can be serious for a person with AD. These drugs should NOT be given to a person with AD. You might talk with the person's doctor about other, safer drugs.

Examples of these drugs include:

- Atrovent® (AT-row-vent), brand name; ipratropium (EYE-pra-troe-pee-um), generic name
- Combivent® (COM-bi-vent), brand name; ipratropium and albuterol (EYE-pra-troe-pee-um and AL-bu-ter-all), generic names
- DuoNeb® (DO-oh-neb), brand name; ipratropium and albuterol (EYE-pra-troe-pee-um and AL-bu-ter-all), generic names
- Spiriva® (SPY-ree-vah), brand name; tiotropium (TEE-oh-tro-pee-um), generic name

Medicines to treat other medical conditions

Many people with AD also have other medical problems such as diabetes, high blood pressure, or heart disease. They may take different medicines for these problems. It's important to track all the medicines they take. Make a list of their medicines and take the list with you when you visit their doctors.

Common Medical Problems in People with AD

A person with AD may have other medical problems over time, as we all do. These problems can cause more confusion and behavior changes. The person may not be able to tell you what is wrong. You need to watch for signs of illness and tell the doctor about what you see.

The most common medical problems

Fever

Having a fever means that the person's temperature is 2 degrees above his or her normal temperature.

A fever may be a sign of:

- Infection, caused by germs
- Dehydration, caused by a lack of fluids
- Heat stroke
- Constipation (discussed later in this section)

Don't use a glass thermometer because the person might bite down on the glass. Use a digital thermometer, which you can buy at a grocery store or drugstore.

Flu and pneumonia

These diseases spread quickly from one person to another, and people with AD are more likely to get them. Make sure that the person gets a flu shot each year and a pneumonia shot once after age 65. Most older people only need the pneumonia shot one time. The shots lower the chances that the person will get flu or pneumonia. For more information on these illnesses, visit the Centers for Disease Control and Prevention website, www.cdc.gov.

MAKE SURE THE PERSON SEES THE DOCTOR

Make sure the person with AD sees a health professional on a regular basis. This is the best thing you can do to help prevent medical problems.

Flu and pneumonia may cause

- Fever (Not everyone with pneumonia has a fever.)
- Chills
- Aches and pains
- Vomiting
- Coughing
- Breathing trouble

Falls

As AD gets worse, the person may have trouble walking and keeping his or her balance. He or she also may have changes in depth perception, which is the ability to understand distances. For example, someone with AD may try to step down when walking from a carpeted to a tile floor. This puts him or her at risk for falls.

To reduce the chance of a fall:

- Clean up clutter.
- Remove throw rugs.
- Use chairs with arms.

- Put grab bars in the bathroom.
- Use good lighting.
- Make sure the person wears sturdy shoes with good traction.

Dehydration

Our bodies must have a certain amount of water to work well. If a person is sick or doesn't drink enough fluid, he or she may become dehydrated.

Signs of dehydration to look for include:

- Dry mouth
- Dizziness
- Hallucinations (Don't forget that hallucinations may be caused by the AD itself.)
- Rapid heart rate

Be aware of how much fluid the person is drinking. This is even more important during hot weather or in homes without air conditioning. Also, look for signs of dehydration during the winter months when heat in your home can create a lot of dry air.

Constipation

People can have constipation—trouble having a bowel movement—when they:

- Change what they eat
- Take certain medicines, including Namenda®
- Get less exercise than usual
- Drink less fluid than usual

Try to get the person to drink at least 6 glasses of liquid a day.

Besides water, other good sources of liquid include:

- Juice, especially prune juice
- Gelatin, such as Jell-O®
- Soup
- Melted ice cream

- Decaffeinated coffee and tea
- Liquid cereal, such as Cream of Wheat®

Have the person eat foods high in fiber. Foods like dried apricots, raisins, or prunes; some dry cereals; or soybeans might help ease constipation.

If possible, make sure that the person gets some exercise each day, such as walking. Call the doctor if you notice a change in the person's bowel habits.

Diarrhea

Some medicines, such as Aricept®, Razadyne®, and Exelon®, may cause diarrhea—loose bowel movements. Certain medical problems also may cause diarrhea. Make sure the person takes in lots of fluids when he or she has diarrhea. Also, be sure to let the doctor know about this problem.

Incontinence

Incontinence means a person can't control his or her bladder and/or bowels. This may happen at any stage of AD, but it is more often a problem in the later stages. Signs of this problem are leaking urine, problems emptying the bladder, and soiled underwear and bed sheets. Be sure to let the doctor know if this happens. He or she may be able to treat the cause of the problem.

Here are some examples of things that can be treated:

- Urinary tract infection
- Enlarged prostate gland
- Too little fluid in the body (dehydration)
- Diabetes that isn't being treated
- Taking too many water pills
- Drinking too much caffeine
- Taking medicines that make it hard to hold urine

When you talk to the doctor, be ready to answer the following questions:

- What medicines is the person taking?
- Does the person leak urine when he or she laughs, coughs, or lifts something?
- Does the person urinate often?
- Can the person get to the bathroom in time?

- Is the person urinating in places other than the bathroom?
- Is the person soiling his or her clothes or bed sheets each night?
- Do these problems happen each day or once in a while?

Here are some ways you can deal with incontinence:

- Remind the person to go to the bathroom every 2 to 3 hours.
- Show him or her the way to the bathroom, or take him or her.
- Make sure that the person wears loose, comfortable clothing that is easy to remove.
- Limit fluids after 6 p.m. if problems happen at night. Do not give the person fluids with caffeine, such as coffee or tea.
- Give the person fresh fruit before bedtime instead of fluids if he or she is thirsty.
- Mark the bathroom door with a big sign that reads "Toilet" or "Bathroom."
- Use a stable toilet seat that is at a good height. Using a colorful toilet seat may help the person identify the toilet. You can buy raised toilet seats at medical supply stores.
- Help the person when he or she needs to use a public bathroom. This may mean going into the stall with the person or using a family or private bathroom.

Things you may want to buy:

- Use adult disposable briefs or underwear, bed protectors, and waterproof mattress covers. You can buy these items at drugstores and medical supply stores.
- Use a drainable pouch for the person who can't control his or her bowel movements. Talk to the nurse about how to use this product.

Some people find it helpful to keep a record of how much food and fluid the person takes in and how often he or she goes to the bathroom. You can use this information to make a schedule of when he or she needs to go to the bathroom.

Dental problems

As AD gets worse, people need help taking care of their teeth or dentures.

Check the person's mouth for any problems such as:

- Sores
- Decayed teeth
- Food "pocketed" in the cheek or on the roof of the mouth
- Lumps

Be sure to take the person for dental checkups. Some people need medicine to calm them before they can see the dentist.

Other medical problems

People with AD can have the same medical problems as many older adults. Research suggests that some of these medical problems may be related to AD.

For example, some heart and blood circulation problems, stroke, and diabetes are more common in people who have AD than in the general population. Diseases caused by infections also are common.

Be sure to take the person to the doctor for regular checkups.

Visiting the doctor

It's important that the person with AD get regular medical care.

Here are some tips to help you get ready for a visit to the doctor's office:

- Make an appointment during the person's best time of day and when the office is not very crowded.
- Let the office staff know before the visit about the person's AD. Ask them for help to make the visit go smoothly.
- Don't tell the person with AD about the visit until the day of the visit or even right before it is time to go if visiting the doctor makes the person nervous. Be positive and matter of fact.
- Take something he or she likes to eat or drink and any materials or activities the person enjoys.
- Have a friend or family member go with you, so that one of you can stay with the person while the other speaks with the doctor.
- Take a brief summary listing the person's medical history, primary care doctor, and current medications.

Going to the emergency room

A trip to the emergency room (ER) can be very stressful for both the person with AD and you.

Here are some ways to cope with ER visits:

- Take a list of medicines, insurance cards, the health care provider's name and phone number, and advance directives. Advance directives are signed documents, such as a living will, that spell out a patient's wishes for end-of-life care.
- Ask a friend or family member to go with you or meet you in the ER. He or she can stay with the person while you answer questions.
- Be ready to explain the symptoms and events leading up to the ER visit. You may have to repeat this more than once to different staff members.
- Tell ER staff that the person has AD. Explain how best to talk with the person.
- If the person with AD must stay overnight in the hospital, try to have a friend or family member stay with him or her.

COPING WITH THE LAST STAGES OF AD

Coping with Late-Stage AD

When a person moves to the later stages of AD, caregiving may become even harder. This section offers ways to cope with changes that take place during severe or late-stage AD.

If caring for the person has become too much for you, see the section on "When You Need Help," for possible sources of help.

When the person with AD can't move

If the person with AD can't move around on his or her own, contact a home health aide, physical therapist, or nurse. Ask the doctor for a referral to one of these health professionals. They can show you how to move the person safely, such as changing his or her position in bed or in a chair. Also, a physical therapist can show you how to move the person's body joints using range-of-motion exercises. During these exercises, you hold the person's arms or legs, one at a time, and move and bend it several times a day. Movement prevents stiffness of the arms, hands, and legs. It also prevents pressure or bedsores.

PAIN ALERT

Always remember that the person with AD may not be able to tell you when he or she is in pain. Watch the person's face to see if it looks like he or she is in pain or feeling ill. Also, notice sudden changes in behavior such as increased yelling or striking out. If you are unsure what to do, call the doctor for help.

How to make someone with AD more comfortable

Here are some ways to make the person with AD more comfortable:

- Buy special mattresses and wedge-shaped seat cushions that reduce pressure sores. You can purchase these at a medical supply store or drugstore or online. Ask the home health aide, nurse, or physical therapist how to use the equipment.
- Move the person to a different position at least every 2 hours.
- Use a lap board to rest the person's arms and support the upper body when he or she is sitting up.
- Give the person something to hold, such as a wash cloth, while being moved. The person will be less likely to grab onto you or the furniture. If he or she is weak on one side, stand on the weak side to support the stronger side and help the person change positions.

How to keep from hurting yourself when moving the person with AD

To keep from hurting yourself when moving someone with AD:

- Know your strength when lifting or moving the person; don't try to do too much. Also, be aware of how you position your body.
- Bend at the knees and then straighten up by using your thigh muscles, not your back.
- Keep your back straight, and don't bend at the waist.

- Hold the person as close as possible to avoid reaching away from your body.
- Place one foot in front of the other, or space your feet comfortably apart for a wide base of support.
- Use little steps to move the person from one seat to another. Don't twist your body.
- Use a transfer or "Posey" belt, shown below. You can buy this belt at a medical supply store or drugstore. To move the person, slide him or her to the edge of the chair or bed by wrapping the transfer belt around the person's waist. Face the person and place your hands under the belt on either side of his or her waist. Then bend your knees, and pull up by using your thigh muscles to raise the person from a seated to a standing position.

How to make sure the person eats well

In the later stages of AD, many people lose interest in food. You may begin to notice some changes in how or when the person eats.

He or she may not:

- Be aware of mealtimes
- Know when he or she has had enough food
- Remember to cook
- Eat enough different kinds of foods

This means the person may not be getting the foods or vitamins and minerals needed to stay healthy. Here are some suggestions to help the person with late-stage AD eat better. Remember that these are just tips. Try different things and see what works best for the person.

You might try to:

- Serve meals at the same time each day.
- Make the eating area quiet. Turn off the TV, CD player, or radio.
- Offer just one food at a time instead of filling the plate or table with too many things.
- Use colorful plates so the person can see the food.

- Control between-meal snacks. Lock the refrigerator door and food cabinets if necessary. Put masking tape near the top and/or bottom of the doors.
- Make sure the person's dentures are tight fitting. Loose dentures or dentures with bumps or cracks may cause choking or pain, making it hard to eat. Take poorly fitting dentures out until the person can get dentures that fit.
- Let the doctor know if your family member loses a lot of weight, for example, if he or she loses 10 pounds in a month.

Here are specific suggestions about foods to eat and liquids to drink:

- Give the person finger foods to eat such as cheese, small sandwiches, small pieces of chicken, fresh fruits, or vegetables. Sandwiches made with pita bread are easier to handle.
- Give him or her high-calorie, healthy foods to eat or drink, such as protein milk shakes. You can buy high-protein drinks and powders at grocery stores, drugstores, or discount stores. Also, you can mix healthy foods in a blender and let the person drink his or her meal. Use diet supplements if he or she is not getting enough calories. Talk with the doctor or nurse about what kinds of supplements are best.
- Try to use healthy fats in cooking, such as olive oil. Also, use extra cooking oil, butter, and mayonnaise to cook and prepare food if the person needs more calories. If the person has heart disease, check with the doctor about how much and what kinds of fat to use.
- If the person has diabetes or high blood pressure, check with the doctor or a nutrition specialist about which foods to limit.
- Have the person take a multivitamin—a tablet, capsule, powder, liquid, or injection that adds vitamins, minerals, and other important things to a person's diet.
- Serve bigger portions at breakfast because it's the first meal of the day.

What to do about swallowing problems

As AD progresses to later stages, the person may no longer be able to chew and swallow easily. This is a serious problem. If the person chokes on each bite of food, there is a chance that the food could go into the lungs. This can cause pneumonia, which can lead to death.

The following suggestions may help with swallowing:

- Make sure you cut the food into small pieces, and make it soft enough to eat.
- Grind food or make it liquid using a blender or baby food grinder.
- Offer soft foods, such as ice cream, milk shakes, yogurt, soups, applesauce, gelatin, or custard.
- Don't use a straw; it may cause more swallowing problems. Instead, have the person drink small sips from a cup.
- Limit the amount of milk the person drinks if it tends to catch in the throat.
- Give the person more cold drinks than hot drinks. Cold drinks are easier to swallow.
- Don't give the person thin liquids, such as coffee, tea, water, or broth, because they are hardest to swallow. You can buy Thick-It® at most pharmacies. You add Thick-It® to liquids to make them thicker. You also can use ice cream and sherbet to thicken liquids.

Here are some other ideas to help people swallow:

- Don't hurry the person. He or she needs time to chew and swallow each mouthful before taking another bite.
- Don't feed a person who is drowsy or lying down. He or she should be in an upright, sitting position during the meal and for at least 20 minutes after the meal.
- Have the person keep his or her neck forward and chin down when swallowing.
- Stroke (gently) the person's neck in a downward motion and say, "swallow" to remind him or her to swallow.
- Find out if the person's pills can be crushed or taken in liquid form.

Helping the person with AD eat can be exhausting. Planning meals ahead and having the food ready can make this task a little easier for you. Also, remember that people with AD may not eat much at certain times and then feel more like eating at other times. It helps to make mealtime as pleasant and enjoyable as possible. But, no matter how well you plan, the person may not be hungry when you're ready to serve food.

Dental, skin, and foot problems

Dental, skin, and foot problems may take place in early and moderate stage AD, but most often happen during late stage AD.

Body jerking

Myoclonus is a condition that sometimes happens with AD. The person's arms, legs, or whole body may jerk. This can look like a seizure, but the person doesn't pass out. Tell the doctor right away if you see these signs. The doctor may prescribe one or more medicines to help reduce symptoms.

Skin problems

Once the person stops walking or stays in one position too long, he or she may get skin or pressure sores.

To prevent skin or pressure sores, you can:

- Move the person at least every 2 hours if he or she is sitting up.
- Move the person at least every hour if he or she is lying down.
- Put a 4-inch foam pad on top of the mattress.
- Check to make sure that the foam pad is comfortable for the person. Some people find these pads too hot for sleeping and may be allergic to them. If the foam pad is a problem, you can get pads filled with gel, air, or water.
- Check to make sure the person sinks a little when lying down on the pad. Also, the pad should fit snugly around his or her body.

To check for pressure sores:

- Look at the person's heels, hips, buttocks, shoulders, back, and elbows for redness or sores.
- Ask the doctor what to do if you find pressure sores.
- Try to keep the person off the affected area.

Foot care

It's important for the person with AD to take care of his or her feet. If the person can't, you will need to do it.

Here's what to do:

- Soak the person's feet in warm water; wash the feet with a mild soap; and check for cuts, corns, and calluses.
- Put lotion on the feet so that the skin doesn't become dry and cracked.
- Cut or file their toenails.
- Talk to a foot care doctor, called a podiatrist, if the person has diabetes or sores on the feet.

End-of-Life Care

Caring for someone in the final stage of life is always hard. It may be even harder when the person has AD. Of course, you want to make the person as comfortable as possible, but he or she can't tell you how. You may become frustrated because you don't know what to do. Also, it can be upsetting because you want the person to talk with you, share memories and feelings, and say goodbye. While the person with AD may not be able to say these things, you can. It's really important to say the things in your heart, whatever helps you to say goodbye.

When the person with AD dies, you may have lots of feelings. You may feel sad, depressed, or angry. You also may feel relieved that the person is no longer suffering and that you don't have to care for the person any longer. Relief sometimes may lead to feelings of guilt. All of these feelings are normal.

Planning for the end of a person's life and knowing what to expect can make this time easier for everyone. Geriatric care managers, grief counselors, and hospice care staff are trained to help you through this time. You might want to contact hospice staff early for help on how to care for the dying person. These professionals can help make the person more comfortable.

END-OF-LIFE CARE

The National Institute on Aging offers helpful information on caregiving, including end-of-life care. Its publications may be ordered free or viewed on the NIA website: www.nia.nih.gov/health

Phone: 1-800-222-2225

CARING FOR YOURSELF

Taking care of yourself is one of the most important things you can do as a caregiver. This could mean asking family members and friends to help out, doing things you enjoy, using adult day care services, or getting help from a local home health care agency. Taking these actions can bring you some relief. It also may help keep you from getting ill or depressed.

How to Take Care of Yourself

Here are some ways you can take care of yourself:

- Ask for help when you need it.
- Join a caregiver's support group.
- Take breaks each day.
- Spend time with friends.
- Keep up with your hobbies and interests.
- Eat healthy foods.
- Get exercise as often as you can.
- See your doctor on a regular basis.
- Keep your health, legal, and financial information up-to-date.

Getting help

Everyone needs help at times. It's okay to ask for help and to take time for yourself. However, many caregivers find it hard to ask for help. You may feel:

- You should be able to do everything yourself
- That it's not all right to leave the person with someone else
- No one will help even if you ask
- You don't have the money to pay someone to watch the person for an hour or two

If you have trouble asking for help, try using some of the tips below.

- It's okay to ask for help from family, friends, and others. I don't have to do everything myself.

- Ask people to help out in specific ways like making a meal, visiting the person, or taking the person out for a short time.
- Join a support group to share advice and understanding with other caregivers.
- Call for help from home health care or adult day care services when you need it.
- Use national and local resources to find out how to pay for some of this help.

AD INFORMATION

You also can call the Alzheimer's Disease Education and Referral Center at no cost. The phone number is 1-800-438-4380. Visit on the Internet at www.nia.nih.gov/alzheimers.

You may want to join a support group of AD caregivers in your area or on the Internet. These groups meet in person or online to share experiences and tips and to give each other support. Ask your doctor, check online, or look in the phone book for a local chapter of the Alzheimer's Association.

If you are a veteran or are caring for one, the Veterans Administration might be of help to you. To learn more, visit their caregivers' website at www.caregiver.va.gov. You might also call their toll-free support line at 1-855-260-3274.

Your emotional health

You may be busy caring for the person with AD and don't take time to think about your emotional health. But, you need to. Caring for a person with AD takes a lot of time and effort. Your job as caregiver can become even harder when the person you're caring for gets angry with you, hurts your feelings, or forgets who you are. Sometimes, you may feel really discouraged, sad, lonely, frustrated, confused, or angry. These feelings are normal.

Here are some things you can say to yourself that might help you feel better:

- I'm doing the best I can.
- What I'm doing would be hard for anyone.
- I'm not perfect, and that's okay.

- I can't control some things that happen.
- Sometimes, I just need to do what works for right now.
- Even when I do everything I can think of, the person with AD will still have problem behaviors because of the illness, not because of what I do.
- I will enjoy the moments when we can be together in peace.
- I will try to get help from a counselor if caregiving becomes too much for me.

Meeting your spiritual needs

Many of us have spiritual needs. Going to a church, temple, or mosque helps some people meet their spiritual needs. They like to be part of a faith community. For others, simply having a sense that larger forces are at work in the world helps meet their spiritual needs. As the caregiver of a person with AD, you may need more spiritual resources than others do.

Meeting your spiritual needs can help you:

- Cope better as a caregiver
- Know yourself and your needs
- Feel recognized, valued, and loved
- Become involved with others
- Find a sense of balance and peace

Other caregivers made these suggestions to help you cope with your feelings and spiritual needs:

- Understand that you may feel powerless and hopeless about what's happening to the person you care for.
- Understand that you may feel a sense of loss and sadness.
- Understand why you've chosen to take care of the person with AD. Ask yourself if you made this choice out of love, loyalty, a sense of duty, a religious obligation, financial concerns, fear, a habit, or self-punishment.
- Let yourself feel day-to-day "uplifts." These might include good feelings about the person you care for, support from other caring people, or time to spend on your own interests and hobbies.

- Keep a connection to something "higher than yourself." This may be a belief in a higher power, religious beliefs, or a belief that something good comes from every life experience.

JOINING A CLINICAL TRIAL

A clinical trial is a research study to find out whether new medicines or other treatments are both safe and effective. Clinical trials most often take place at research centers and universities across the United States. Joining a clinical trial, also called a research study, is a way for you and the person with AD to help find ways to prevent or treat AD.

A clinical trial gives the person a chance to get a new treatment from researchers, before the government approves it. The new treatment might be a new medicine or a new way to care for someone with AD. A clinical trial is another way to get care from experts. Being in a study also gives you and the person with AD a chance to help others who have the disease. But, you should keep in mind that clinical trials may have some risks. Be sure to look at the benefits and risks of a clinical trial before you make your decision.

How Can a Person Join a Clinical Trial?

To join, you first must find a study that is looking for people like you or the person with AD. For more information about AD clinical trials and studies, visit the ADEAR Center Clinical Trials Database at www.nia.nih.gov/alzheimers/clinical-trials. You can also call 1-800-438-4380. An information specialist can help you look for a clinical trial.

You may also want to visit these clinical trials websites:

- Alzheimer's Association www.alz.org/alzheimers_disease_clinical_studies.asp
- National Institutes of Health
  www.nih.gov/health/clinicaltrials
  www.clinicaltrials.gov
- Alzheimer's Disease Cooperative Study
  www.adcs.org

What Else Do I Need to Know about Clinical Trials?

The government has strict rules to protect the safety and privacy of people in clinical trials. The researchers conducting the study are required by law to tell the patient and/or family members all of the risks and benefits of taking part in the study. This is called the informed consent process. As part of this process, the person reads an informed consent form. The form explains the study, its risks and benefits, and the rights of the person taking part in the study. The laws and rules about informed consent differ across States and research centers.

Some clinical trials will pay you back for transportation costs, child care, meals, and lodging; others won't. Talk with the study coordinator about these costs.

Call the ADEAR Center at 1-800-438-4380 or go to www.nia.nih.gov/alzheimers for free information on participating in Alzheimer's disease clinical trials and studies.

SUMMARY

Thank you for reading this chapter. We hope it helps you— the caregiver—and the person with AD.

Here are some main points to remember:

- Learn about AD to help you cope with challenges.
- Plan how to care for someone with AD to make things easier.
- Create a safe home for the person with AD.
- It's important for you to take care of yourself as well as the person with AD.
- You aren't alone. It's okay to ask for and get help. Check the resources listed in this book.
- You can find the right place for the person with AD if he or she can no longer live at home.
- Learn about medicines used for people with AD.
- Find out how to cope with late-stage AD.

WORDS TO KNOW

Aggression (uh-GRESH-un). When a person lashes out verbally or tries to hit or hurt someone.

Agitation (aj-uh-TAY-shun). Restlessness and worry that some people with AD feel. Agitation may cause pacing, sleeplessness, or aggression.

Alzheimer's disease (AD) (ALLZ-high-merz duh-ZEEZ). Disease that causes large numbers of nerve cells in the brain to die. People with AD lose the ability to remember, think, and make good judgments. At some point, they will need full-time care.

Anti-anxiety (an-tye-ang-ZYE-eh-tee) **drugs**. Drugs used to treat agitation and extreme worry. Some can cause sleepiness, falls, and confusion. These drugs should be taken with caution.

Anticholinergic (an-tye-KOL-in-er-gik) **drugs**. Drugs used to treat stomach cramps, incontinence, asthma, motion sickness, and muscle spasms. **These drugs should not be given to people with AD.**

Anticonvulsants (an-tye-kon-VUL-sunts). Drugs sometimes used to treat severe aggression.

Antidepressants (an-tye-dee-PRESS-unts). Drugs used to reduce depression and worry.

Antipsychotics (an-tye-sye-KOT-iks). Drugs used to treat paranoia, hallucinations, sleeplessness, agitation, aggression, and other personality and behavior disorders. These drugs should be taken with caution.

Assisted living facility. Type of living facility that provides rooms or apartments for people who can handle most of their own care, but may need some help.

Caregiver. Anyone who takes care of a person with AD.

Clinical trial. Research study to find out whether new medicines or other treatments are both safe and effective.

Constipation (kon-sti-PAY-shun). Trouble having a bowel movement.

Continuing care retirement community. Community of homes, apartments, and rooms that offer different levels of care for older people.

Deductible (dee-DUK-ti-bul). The amount of medical expenses that a person must pay per year before the insurance company will cover medical costs.

Dehydration (dee-hye-DRAY-shun). Condition caused by lack of fluids in the body.

Delusions (duh-LOO-zhuhns). False beliefs that someone with AD believes are real.

Diarrhea (dye-uh-REE-uh). Loose bowel movements.

Do Not Resuscitate (DNR) Form. Document that tells health care staff how the person with AD wants end-of-life health care managed.

Durable Power of Attorney for Finances. Legal permission for someone to make legal and financial decisions for the person with AD, after he or she no longer can.

Durable Power of Attorney for Health Care. Legal permission for someone to make health care decisions for the person with AD, after he or she no longer can.

Hallucinations (huh-loo-suh-NAY-shuns). One possible effect of AD, in which the person sees, hears, smells, tastes, and/or feels something that isn't there.

Home health care. Service that provides care and/or companionship in the home for the person with AD.

Hospice services. Services that provide care for a person who is near the end of life and support for families during this time.

Hypersexuality (hi-pur-sek-shoo-AL-uh-tee). Condition in which people with AD become overly interested in sex.

Incontinence (in-KON-ti-nunts). Trouble controlling bladder and/or bowels.

Inpatient facility. Hospital or other medical facility where people stay in the facility.

Intimacy. Special bond between people who love and respect each other.

Living trust. Legal document that tells a person called a trustee how to distribute a person's property and money.

Living will. Legal document that states a person's wishes for end-of-life health care.

Multivitamin (mull-tee-VYE-tuh-min). A tablet, capsule, powder, liquid, or injection that adds vitamins, minerals, and other nutritional elements to the diet.

Myoclonus (mye-o-KLO-nuss). Condition that sometimes happens with AD, in which a person's arms, legs, or whole body may jerk. It can look like a seizure, but the person doesn't pass out.

Nursing home. Home for people who can't care for themselves anymore. Some have special AD care units.

Paranoia (pare-uh-NOY-uh). Type of delusion in which a person believes—without good reason—that others are being unfair, unfriendly, or dishonest. Paranoia may cause suspicion, fear, or jealousy in a person with AD.

Sexuality. Important way that people express their feelings physically and emotionally for one another.

Spirituality (SPEAR-uh-choo-al-ity). Belief in a higher power or in larger forces at work in the world. Going to church, temple, or mosque helps some people meet their spiritual needs. For others, simply having a sense that larger forces are at work in the world helps meet their spiritual needs.

Sundowning. Restlessness in a person with AD that usually starts around dinnertime or in the evening and may make it hard to get the person to go to bed and stay there.

Urinary tract infection (YUR-in-air-ee tract in-FEK-shun). An illness, usually in the bladder or kidneys, caused by bacteria in the urine.

Will. Legal document that tells how a person's money and property will be divided after his or her death.

In: Alzheimer's Disease: A Caregivers Guide ISBN: 978-1-63117-720-0
Editor: Diana B. Watkins

Chapter 2

HOME SAFETY FOR PEOPLE WITH ALZHEIMER'S DISEASE*

National Institute on Aging

INTRODUCTION

Caring for a person with Alzheimer's disease is a challenge that calls upon the patience, creativity, knowledge, and skills of each caregiver. We hope that this chapter will help you cope with some of these challenges and develop creative solutions to increase the security and freedom of the person with Alzheimer's in your home, as well as your own peace of mind.

This chapter is for those who provide in-home care for people with Alzheimer's disease or related disorders. Our goal is to improve home safety by identifying potential problems in the home and offering possible solutions to help prevent accidents.

We begin with a checklist to help you make each room in your home a safer environment for the person with Alzheimer's. Next, we hope to increase awareness of the ways specific impairments associated with the disease can create particular safety hazards in the home. Home safety tips are listed to help you cope with some of the more hazardous behaviors that may occur as the disease advances. We also include tips for managing driving and planning for

* This is an edited, reformatted and augmented version of NIH Publication No. 02-5179, dated August 2010.

natural disaster safety. The chapter ends with a list of resources for family caregivers.

What Is Alzheimer's Disease?

Alzheimer's disease is a progressive, irreversible brain disease that slowly destroys memory and thinking skills. Estimates vary, but experts suggest that as many as 5.1 million Americans have the disease, which affects people of all racial, economic, and educational backgrounds. Although Alzheimer's primarily affects people age 60 or older, it also may affect people in their 50s and, rarely, even younger.

Alzheimer's disease is the most common cause of dementia in adults. Dementia is a loss of memory and intellect that interferes with daily life and activities. Dementia is not a disease; rather, it is a group of symptoms that may accompany certain diseases and conditions. Other symptoms include changes in personality, mood, or behavior.

Other causes of irreversible dementia include vascular dementia and alcohol abuse. The recommendations in this chapter deal primarily with common problems in Alzheimer's, but they also may be helpful for people with other types of dementia.

What Are the Symptoms of Alzheimer's Disease?

There is no "typical" person with Alzheimer's disease. There is tremendous variability among people with Alzheimer's in their behaviors and symptoms. At present, there is no way to predict how quickly the disease will progress in any one person or the exact changes that will occur. We do know, however, that many of these changes will present problems for caregivers. Therefore, knowledge and prevention are critical to safety.

People with Alzheimer's disease have memory problems and cognitive impairment (difficulties with thinking and reasoning), and eventually they will not be able to care for themselves. They often experience confusion, loss of judgment, and difficulty finding words, finishing thoughts, or following directions. They also may experience personality and behavior changes. For example, they may become agitated, irritable, or very passive. Some people with Alzheimer's wander from home and become lost. Others may not be able to tell the difference between day and night—they may wake up, get dressed, and start to leave the house in the middle of the night, thinking that the day has just started. People with Alzheimer's also can have losses that affect vision, smell, or taste.

These disabilities are very difficult, not only for the person with Alzheimer's, but for the caregiver, family, and other loved ones as well. Caregivers need resources and reassurance to know that while the challenges are great, specific actions can reduce some of the safety concerns that accompany Alzheimer's disease.

General Safety Concerns

People with Alzheimer's disease become increasingly unable to take care of themselves. However, the disease progresses differently in each person. As a caregiver, you face the ongoing challenge of adapting to each change in the person's behavior and functioning. The following general principles may be helpful.

1. **Think prevention.** It is very difficult to predict what a person with Alzheimer's might do. Just because something has not yet occurred does not mean it should not be cause for concern. Even with the best-laid plans, accidents can happen. Therefore, checking the safety of your home will help you take control of some of the potential problems that may create hazardous situations.
2. **Adapt the environment.** It is more effective to change the environment than to change most behaviors. While some Alzheimer's behaviors can be managed with special medications prescribed by a doctor, many cannot. You can make changes in an environment to decrease the hazards and stressors that accompany these behavioral and functional changes.
3. **Minimize danger.** By minimizing danger, you can maximize independence. A safe environment can be a less restrictive environment where the person with Alzheimer's disease can experience increased security and more mobility.

Is It Safe to Leave the Person with Alzheimer's Disease Alone?

This issue needs careful evaluation and is certainly a safety concern. The following points may help you decide.

Does the person with Alzheimer's:

- become confused or unpredictable under stress?
- recognize a dangerous situation, such as fire?
- know how to use the telephone in an emergency?
- know how to get help?
- stay content within the home?
- wander and become disoriented?
- show signs of agitation, depression, or withdrawal when left alone for any period of time?
- attempt to pursue former interests or hobbies that might now warrant supervision, such as cooking, appliance repair, or woodworking?

You may want to seek input and advice from a health care professional to assist you in these considerations. As Alzheimer's disease progresses, these questions will need ongoing evaluation.

Home Safety Room by Room

Prevention begins with a safety check of every room in your home. Use the following room-by-room checklist to alert you to potential hazards and to record any changes you need to make. You can buy products or gadgets necessary for home safety at stores carrying hardware, electronics, medical supplies, and children's items.

Keep in mind that it may not be necessary to make all of the suggested changes. This chapter covers a wide range of safety concerns that may arise, and some modifications may never be needed. It is important, however, to re-evaluate home safety periodically as behavior and abilities change.

Your home is a personal and precious environment. As you go through this checklist, some of the changes you make may impact your surroundings positively, and some may affect you in ways that may be inconvenient or undesirable. It is possible, however, to strike a balance. Caregivers can make adaptations that modify and simplify without severely disrupting the home. You may want to consider setting aside a special area for yourself, a space off-limits to anyone else and arranged exactly as you like. Everyone needs private, quiet time, and as a caregiver, this becomes especially crucial.

A safe home can be a less stressful home for the person with Alzheimer's disease, the caregiver, and family members. You don't have to make these changes alone. You may want to enlist the help of a friend, professional, or community service such as the Alzheimer's Association.

Throughout the Home

- Display emergency numbers and your home address near all telephones.
- Use an answering machine when you cannot answer phone calls, and set it to turn on after the fewest number of rings possible. A person with Alzheimer's disease often may be unable to take messages or could become a victim of telephone exploitation. Turn ringers on low to avoid distraction and confusion. Put all portable and cell phones and equipment in a safe place so they will not be easily lost.
- Install smoke alarms and carbon monoxide detectors in or near the kitchen and all sleeping areas. Check their functioning and batteries frequently.
- Avoid the use of flammable and volatile compounds near gas appliances. Do not store these materials in an area where a gas pilot light is used.
- Install secure locks on all outside doors and windows.
- Hide a spare house key outside in case the person with Alzheimer's locks you out of the house.
- Avoid the use of extension cords if possible by placing lamps and appliances close to electrical outlets. Tack extension cords to the baseboards of a room to avoid tripping.
- Cover unused electrical outlets with childproof plugs.

- Place red tape around floor vents, radiators, and other heating devices to deter the person with Alzheimer's from standing on or touching them when hot.
- Check all rooms for adequate lighting.
- Place light switches at the top and the bottom of stairs.
- Stairways should have at least one handrail that extends beyond the first and last steps. If possible, stairways should be carpeted or have safety grip strips. Put a gate across the stairs if the person has balance problems.
- Keep all medications (prescription and over-the-counter) locked. Each bottle of prescription medicine should be clearly labeled with the person's name, name of the drug, drug strength, dosage frequency, and expiration date. Child-resistant caps are available if needed.
- Keep all alcohol in a locked cabinet or out of reach of the person with Alzheimer's. Drinking alcohol can increase confusion.
- If smoking is permitted, monitor the person with Alzheimer's while he or she is smoking. Remove matches, lighters, ashtrays, cigarettes, and other means of smoking from view. This reduces fire hazards, and with these reminders out of sight, the person may forget the desire to smoke.
- Avoid clutter, which can create confusion and danger. Throw out or recycle newspapers and magazines regularly. Keep all areas where people walk free of furniture.
- Keep plastic bags out of reach. A person with Alzheimer's disease may choke or suffocate.
- Remove all guns and other weapons from the home or lock them up. Install safety locks on guns or remove ammunition and firing pins.
- Lock all power tools and machinery in the garage, workroom, or basement.
- Remove all poisonous plants from the home. Check with local nurseries or contact the poison control center (1-800-222-1222) for a list of poisonous plants.
- Make sure all computer equipment and accessories, including electrical cords, are kept out of the way. If valuable documents or materials are stored on a home computer, protect the files with passwords and back up the files. Password protect access to the

Internet, and restrict the amount of online time without supervision. Consider monitoring computer use by the person with Alzheimer's, and install software that screens for objectionable or offensive material on the Internet.

- Keep fish tanks out of reach. The combination of glass, water, electrical pumps, and potentially poisonous aquatic life could be harmful to a curious person with Alzheimer's disease.

Outside Approaches to the House

- Keep steps sturdy and textured to prevent falls in wet or icy weather.
- Mark the edges of steps with bright or reflective tape.
- Consider installing a ramp with handrails as an alternative to steps.
- Eliminate uneven surfaces or walkways, hoses, and other objects that may cause a person to trip.
- Restrict access to a swimming pool by fencing it with a locked gate, covering it, and closely supervising it when in use.
- In the patio area, remove the fuel source and fire starters from any grills when not in use, and supervise use when the person with Alzheimer's is present.
- Place a small bench or table by the entry door to hold parcels while unlocking the door.
- Make sure outside lighting is adequate. Light sensors that turn on lights automatically as you approach the house may be useful. They also may be used in other parts of the home.
- Prune bushes and foliage well away from walkways and doorways.
- Consider a NO SOLICITING sign for the front gate or door.

Entryway

- Remove scatter rugs and throw rugs.
- Use textured strips or nonskid wax on hardwood and tile floors to prevent slipping.

Kitchen

- Install childproof door latches on storage cabinets and drawers designated for breakable or dangerous items. Lock away all household cleaning products, matches, knives, scissors, blades, small appliances, and anything valuable.
- If prescription or nonprescription drugs are kept in the kitchen, store them in a locked cabinet.
- Remove scatter rugs and foam pads from the floor.
- Install safety knobs and an automatic shut-off switch on the stove.
- Do not use or store flammable liquids in the kitchen. Lock them in the garage or in an outside storage unit.
- Keep a night-light in the kitchen.
- Remove or secure the family "junk drawer." A person with Alzheimer's may eat small items such as matches, hardware, erasers, and plastics.
- Remove artificial fruits and vegetables or food-shaped kitchen magnets, which might appear to be edible.
- Insert a drain trap in the kitchen sink to catch anything that may otherwise become lost or clog the plumbing.
- Consider disconnecting the garbage disposal. People with Alzheimer's may place objects or their own hands in the disposal.

Bedroom

- Anticipate the reasons a person with Alzheimer's disease might get out of bed, such as hunger, thirst, going to the bathroom, restlessness, and pain. Try to meet these needs by offering food and fluids and scheduling ample toileting.
- Use a night-light.
- Use a monitoring device (like those used for infants) to alert you to any sounds indicating a fall or other need for help. This also is an effective device for bathrooms.
- Remove scatter rugs and throw rugs.
- Remove portable space heaters. If you use portable fans, be sure that objects cannot be placed in the blades.

- Be cautious when using electric mattress pads, electric blankets, electric sheets, and heating pads, all of which can cause burns and fires. Keep controls out of reach.
- If the person with Alzheimer's disease is at risk of falling out of bed, place mats next to the bed, as long as they do not create a greater risk of accident.
- Use transfer or mobility aids.
- If you are considering using a hospital-type bed with rails and/or wheels, read the Food and Drug Administration's up-to-date safety information at www.fda.gov/cdrh/beds.

Bathroom

- Do not leave a severely impaired person with Alzheimer's alone in the bathroom.
- Remove the lock from the bathroom door to prevent the person with Alzheimer's from getting locked inside.
- Place nonskid adhesive strips, decals, or mats in the tub and shower. If the bathroom is uncarpeted, consider placing these strips next to the tub, toilet, and sink.
- Use washable wall-to-wall bathroom carpeting to prevent slipping on wet tile floors.
- Use a raised toilet seat with handrails, or install grab bars beside the toilet.
- Install grab bars in the tub/shower. A grab bar in contrasting color to the wall is easier to see.
- Use a foam rubber faucet cover (often used for small children) in the tub to prevent serious injury should the person with Alzheimer's disease fall.
- Use a plastic shower stool and a handheld shower head to make bathing easier.
- In the shower, tub, and sink, use a single faucet that mixes hot and cold water to avoid burns.
- Set the water heater at 120 degrees Fahrenheit to avoid scalding tap water.
- Insert drain traps in sinks to catch small items that may be lost or flushed down the drain.

- Store medications (prescription and nonprescription) in a locked cabinet. Check medication dates and throw away outdated medications.
- Remove cleaning products from under the sink, or lock them away.
- Use a night-light.
- Remove small electrical appliances from the bathroom. Cover electrical outlets.
- If a man with Alzheimer's disease uses an use electric razor, have him use a mirror outside the bathroom to avoid water contact.

Living Room

- Clear electrical cords from all areas where people walk.
- Remove scatter rugs and throw rugs. Repair or replace torn carpet.
- Place decals at eye level on sliding glass doors, picture windows, and furniture with large glass panels to identify the glass pane.
- Do not leave the person with Alzheimer's disease alone with an open fire in the fireplace. Consider alternative heating sources.
- Keep matches and cigarette lighters out of reach.
- Keep the remote controls for the television, DVD player, and stereo system out of sight.

Laundry Room

- Keep the door to the laundry room locked if possible.
- Lock all laundry products in a cabinet.
- Remove large knobs from the washer and dryer if the person with Alzheimer's tampers with machinery.
- Close and latch the doors and lids to the washer and dryer to prevent objects from being placed in the machines.

Garage/Shed/Basement

- Lock access to all garages, sheds, and basements if possible.

- Inside a garage or shed, keep all potentially dangerous items, such as tools, tackle, machines, and sporting equipment, either locked away in cabinets or in appropriate boxes or cases.
- Secure and lock all motor vehicles and keep them out of sight if possible. Consider covering vehicles, including bicycles, that are not frequently used. This may reduce the possibility that the person with Alzheimer's will think about leaving.
- Keep all toxic materials, such as paint, fertilizers, gasoline, or cleaning supplies, out of view. Either put them in a high, dry place, or lock them in a cabinet.
- If the person with Alzheimer's is permitted in a garage, shed, or basement, preferably with supervision, make sure the area is well lit and that stairs have a handrail and are safe to walk up and down. Keep walkways clear of debris and clutter, and place overhanging items out of reach.

HOME SAFETY BEHAVIOR BY BEHAVIOR

Although a number of behavior and sensory problems may accompany Alzheimer's disease, not every person will experience the disease in exactly the same way. As the disease progresses, particular behavioral changes can create safety problems. The person with Alzheimer's may or may not have these symptoms. However, should these behaviors occur, the following safety recommendations may help reduce risks.

Wandering

- Remove clutter and clear the pathways from room to room to prevent falls and allow the person with Alzheimer's to move about more freely.
- Make sure floors provide good traction for walking or pacing. Use nonskid floor wax or leave floors unpolished. Secure all rug edges, eliminate throw rugs, or install nonskid strips. The person with Alzheimer's should wear nonskid shoes or sneakers.

- Place locks high or low on exit doors so they are out of direct sight. Consider installing double locks that require a key. Keep a key for yourself, and hide one near the door for emergency exit purposes.
- Use loosely fitting doorknob covers so that the cover turns instead of the actual knob. *Due to the potential hazard they could cause if an emergency exit is needed, locked doors and doorknob covers should be used only when a caregiver is present.*
- Install safety devices found in hardware stores to limit how much windows can be opened.
- If possible, secure the yard with fencing and a locked gate. Use door alarms such as loose bells above the door or devices that ring when the doorknob is touched or the door is opened.
- Divert the attention of the person with Alzheimer's disease away from using the door by placing small scenic posters on the door; placing removable gates, curtains, or brightly colored streamers across the door; or wallpapering the door to match any adjoining walls.
- Place STOP, DO NOT ENTER, or CLOSED signs on doors in strategic areas.
- Keep shoes, keys, suitcases, coats, hats, and other signs of departure out of sight.
- Obtain a medical identification bracelet for the person with Alzheimer's with the words "memory loss" inscribed along with an emergency phone number. Place the bracelet on the person's dominant hand to limit the possibility of removal, or solder the bracelet closed. Check with the local Alzheimer's Association about the Safe Return program.
- Place labels in garments to aid in identification.
- Keep an article of the person's worn, unwashed clothing in a plastic bag to aid in finding someone with the use of dogs.
- Notify neighbors of the person's potential to wander or become lost. Alert them to contact you or the police immediately if the individual is seen alone and on the move.
- Give local police, neighbors, and relatives a recent photo of the person with Alzheimer's, along with the person's name and pertinent information, as a precaution should he or she become lost. Keep extra photos on hand.
- Consider making an up-to-date home video of the person with Alzheimer's disease.

- Do not leave a person with Alzheimer's who has a history of wandering unattended.

Rummaging/Hiding Things

- Lock up all dangerous or toxic products, or place them out of the person's reach.
- Remove all old or spoiled food from the refrigerator and cupboards. A person with Alzheimer's may rummage for snacks but may lack the judgment or taste to rule out spoiled foods.
- Simplify the environment by removing clutter or valuable items that could be misplaced, lost, or hidden by the person with Alzheimer's disease. These include important papers, checkbooks, charge cards, and jewelry.
- If your yard has a fence with a locked gate, place the mailbox outside the gate. People with Alzheimer's often hide, lose, or throw away mail. If this is a serious problem, consider obtaining a post office box.
- Create a special place for the person with Alzheimer's to rummage freely or sort (for example, a chest of drawers, a bag of selected objects, or a basket of clothing to fold or unfold). Often, safety problems occur when the person with Alzheimer's becomes bored or does not know what to do.
- Provide the person with Alzheimer's a safe box, treasure chest, or cupboard to store special objects.
- Close access to unused rooms, thereby limiting the opportunity for rummaging and hiding things.
- Search the house periodically to discover hiding places. Once found, these hiding places can be discreetly and frequently checked.
- Keep all trash cans covered or out of sight. The person with Alzheimer's disease may not remember the purpose of the container or may rummage through it.
- Check trash containers before emptying them in case something has been hidden there or accidentally thrown away.

Hallucinations, Illusions, and Delusions

Due to complex changes occurring in the brain, people with Alzheimer's may see or hear things that have no basis in reality. *Hallucinations* involve hearing, seeing, smelling, or feeling things that are not really there. For example, a person with Alzheimer's may see children playing in the living room when no children are there. *Illusions* differ from hallucinations because the person with Alzheimer's is misinterpreting something that actually does exist. Shadows on the wall may look like people, for example. *Delusions* are false beliefs that the person thinks are real. For example, stealing may be suspected but cannot be verified.

It is important to seek medical evaluation if a person with Alzheimer's has ongoing disturbing hallucinations, illusions, or delusions. Discuss with the doctor any illnesses the person has and medicines he or she is taking. An illness or medicine may cause hallucinations or delusions. Often, these symptoms can be treated with medication or behavior management techniques. With all of these symptoms, the following environmental adaptations also may be helpful.

- Paint walls a light color to reflect more light. Use solid colors, which to an impaired person are less confusing than a patterned wall. Large, bold prints (for example, florals in wallpaper or drapes) may cause confusing illusions.
- Make sure there is adequate lighting and keep extra bulbs handy in a secured place. Dimly lit areas may produce confusing shadows or difficulty with interpreting everyday objects.
- Reduce glare by using soft light or frosted bulbs, partially closing blinds or curtains, and maintaining adequate globes or shades on light fixtures.
- Remove or cover mirrors if they cause the person with Alzheimer's disease to become confused or frightened.
- Ask if the person can point to a specific area that is producing confusion. Perhaps one particular aspect of the environment is being misinterpreted.
- Vary the home environment as little as possible to minimize the potential for visual confusion. Keep furniture in the same place.
- Avoid violent or disturbing television programs. The person with Alzheimer's may believe a story is real.

- Do not confront the person with Alzheimer's who becomes aggressive. Withdraw and make sure you have access to an exit as needed.

SPECIAL OCCASIONS/GATHERINGS/HOLIDAYS

When celebrations, special events, or holidays include large numbers of people, remember that large groups may cause a person with Alzheimer's disease some confusion and anxiety. The person with Alzheimer's may find some situations easier and more pleasurable than others.

- Large gatherings, weddings, family reunions, or picnics may cause anxiety. Consider having a more intimate gathering with only a few people in your home. Think about having friends and family visit in small groups rather than all at once. If you are hosting a large group, remember to prepare the person with Alzheimer's ahead of time. Try to have a space available where he or she can rest, be alone, or spend some time with a smaller number of people, if needed.
- Consider simplifying your holidays around the home, and remember that you already may have more responsibilities than in previous years. For example, rather than cooking an elaborate dinner at Thanksgiving or Christmas, invite family and friends for a potluck dinner. Instead of elaborate decorations, consider choosing a few select items to celebrate holidays. Make sure holiday decorations do not significantly alter the environment, which might confuse the person with Alzheimer's disease.
- Holiday decorations, such as Christmas trees, lights, or menorahs, should be secured so that they do not fall or catch on fire. Anything flammable should be monitored at all times, and extra precautions should be taken so that lights or breakable items are fixed firmly, correctly, and out of the way of those with Alzheimer's disease.
- As suggested by most manufacturers, candles of any size should never be lit without supervision. When not in use, they should be put away.
- Try to avoid clutter in general, especially in walkways, during the holidays.

Impairment of the Senses

Alzheimer's disease can cause changes in a person's ability to interpret what he or she can see, hear, taste, feel, or smell. The person with Alzheimer's should be evaluated periodically by a physician for any such changes that may be correctable with glasses, dentures, hearing aids, or other devices.

Vision

People with Alzheimer's may experience a number of changes in visual abilities. For example, they may lose their ability to comprehend visual images. Although there is nothing physically wrong with their eyes, people with Alzheimer's may no longer be able to interpret accurately what they see because of brain changes. Also, their sense of perception and depth may be altered. These changes can cause safety concerns.

- Create color contrast between floors and walls to help the person see depth. Floor coverings are less visually confusing if they are a solid color.
- Use dishes and placemats in contrasting colors for easier identification.
- Mark the edges of steps with brightly colored strips of tape to outline changes in height.
- Place brightly colored signs or simple pictures on doors to important rooms (the bathroom, for example) for easier identification.
- Be aware that a small pet that blends in with the floor or lies in walkways may be a hazard. The person with Alzheimer's disease may trip over the pet.

Smell

A loss of or decrease in the sense of smell often accompanies Alzheimer's disease.

- Install smoke detectors and check them frequently. The person with Alzheimer's disease may not smell smoke or may not associate it with danger.
- Keep refrigerators clear of spoiled foods.

Touch

People with Alzheimer's may experience loss of sensation or may no longer be able to interpret feelings of heat, cold, or discomfort.

- Set water heaters at 120 degrees Fahrenheit to avoid scalding tap water. Most hot water heaters are set at 150 degrees, which can cause burns.
- Color code separate water faucet handles, with red for hot and blue for cold.
- Place a sign on the oven, coffee maker, toaster, crock-pot, iron, and other potentially hot appliances that says DO NOT TOUCH or STOP! VERY HOT. The person with Alzheimer's should not use appliances without supervision. Unplug appliances when not in use.
- Use a thermometer to tell you if bath water is too hot or too cold.
- Remove furniture or other objects with sharp corners or pad the corners to reduce potential for injury.

Taste

People with Alzheimer's disease may lose taste sensitivity. As their judgment declines, they also may place dangerous or inappropriate things in their mouths.

- Keep all condiments such as salt, sugar, or spices hidden if you see the person with Alzheimer's using excess amounts. Too much salt, sugar, or spice can be irritating to the stomach or cause other health problems.
- Remove or lock up medicine cabinet items such as toothpaste, perfume, lotions, shampoos, rubbing alcohol, and soap, which may look and smell like food to the person with Alzheimer's.

- Consider a childproof latch on the refrigerator, if necessary.
- Keep the toll-free poison control number (1-800-222-1222) by the telephone. Keep a bottle of ipecac (vomit-inducing agent) available, but use only with instructions from poison control or 911.
- Keep pet litter boxes inaccessible to the person with Alzheimer's disease. Do not store pet food in the refrigerator.
- Learn the Heimlich maneuver or other techniques to use in case of choking. Check with your local Red Cross chapter for more information and instruction.
- If possible, keep a spare set of dentures. If the person keeps removing dentures, check for correct fit.

Hearing

People with Alzheimer's disease may have normal hearing, but they may lose their ability to interpret what they hear accurately. This loss may result in confusion or overstimulation.

- Avoid excessive noise in the home such as having the stereo and the TV on at the same time.
- Be sensitive to the amount of noise outside the home, and close windows or doors, if necessary.
- Avoid large gatherings of people in the home if the person with Alzheimer's shows signs of agitation or distress in crowds.
- If the person wears a hearing aid, check the batteries and functioning often.

DRIVING

Driving is a complex activity that demands quick reactions, alert senses, and split-second decisionmaking. For a person with Alzheimer's disease, driving becomes increasingly difficult. Memory loss, impaired judgment, disorientation, impaired visual and spatial perception, slow reaction time, certain medications, diminished attention span, and inability to recognize cues such as stop signs and traffic lights can make driving particularly hazardous.

People with Alzheimer's who continue to drive can be a danger to themselves, their passengers, and the community at large. As the disease progresses, they lose driving skills and must stop driving. Unfortunately, people with Alzheimer's often cannot recognize when they should no longer drive. This is a tremendous safety concern. It is extremely important to have the impaired person's driving abilities carefully evaluated.

Explaining to the person with Alzheimer's disease that he or she can no longer drive can be extremely difficult. Loss of driving privileges may represent a tremendous loss of independence, freedom, and identity. It is a significant concern for the person with Alzheimer's and the caregiver. The issue of not driving may produce anger, denial, and grief in the person with Alzheimer's, as well as guilt and anxiety in the caregiver. Family and concerned professionals need to be both sensitive and firm. Above all, they should be persistent and consistent.

The doctor of a person with Alzheimer's disease can assist the family with the task of restricting driving. Talk with the doctor about your concerns. Most people will listen to their doctor. Ask the doctor to advise the person with Alzheimer's to reduce his or her driving, go for a driving evaluation or test, or stop driving altogether. An increasing number of States have laws requiring physicians to report Alzheimer's and related disorders to the Department of Motor Vehicles. The Department of Motor Vehicles then is responsible for retesting the at-risk driver. Testing should occur regularly, at least yearly.

When dementia impairs driving and the person with Alzheimer's disease continues to insist on driving, a number of different approaches may be necessary.

- Work as a team with family, friends, and professionals, and use a single, simple explanation for the loss of driving ability such as: "You have a memory problem, and it is no longer safe to drive," "You cannot drive because you are on medication," or "The doctor has prescribed that you no longer drive."
- Ask the doctor to write on a prescription pad DO NOT DRIVE. Ask the doctor to write to the Department of Motor Vehicles or Department of Public Safety saying this person should no longer drive. Show the letter to the person with Alzheimer's disease as evidence.
- Offer to drive, or ask a friend or family member to drive.
- Walk when possible, and make these outings special events.

- Use public transportation or any special transportation provided by community organizations. Ask about senior discounts or transportation coupons. The person with Alzheimer's should not take public transportation unsupervised.
- Park the car at a friend's home.
- Hide the car keys.
- Exchange car keys with a set of unusable keys. Some people with Alzheimer's are in the habit of carrying keys.
- Place a large note under the car hood requesting that any mechanic call you before doing work requested by the person with Alzheimer's disease.
- Have a mechanic install a "kill switch" or alarm system that disengages the fuel line to prevent the car from starting.
- Consider selling the car and putting aside for taxi fares the money saved from insurance, repairs, and gasoline.
- Do not leave a person with Alzheimer's alone in a parked car.

Warning Signs of Unsafe Driving

Often, the caregiver or a family member, neighbor, or friend is the first to become aware of the safety hazards of someone with Alzheimer's behind the wheel. If the driver with Alzheimer's disease experiences one or more of the following problems, it may be time to limit or stop driving.

Does the person with Alzheimer's:

- get lost while driving in a familiar location?
- fail to observe traffic signals?
- drive at an inappropriate speed?
- become angry, frustrated, or confused while driving?
- make slow or poor decisions?

Please do not wait for an accident to happen. Take action immediately!

Natural Disaster Safety

Natural disasters come in many forms and degrees of severity. They seldom give warning, and they call upon good judgment and the ability to follow through with crisis plans. People with Alzheimer's disease are at a serious disadvantage. Their impairments in memory and reasoning severely limit their ability to act appropriately in crises.

It is always important to have a plan of action in case of fire, earthquake, flood, tornado, or other disasters. Specific home safety precautions may apply and environmental changes may be needed. The American Red Cross is an excellent resource for general safety information and preparedness guides for comprehensive planning. If there is a person with Alzheimer's in the home, the following precautions apply:

- Get to know the neighbors, and identify specific individuals who would be willing to help in a crisis. Formulate a plan of action with them should the person with Alzheimer's be unattended during a crisis.
- Give neighbors a list of emergency phone numbers of caregivers, family members, and primary medical resources.
- Educate neighbors beforehand about the person's specific disabilities, including inability to follow complex instructions, memory loss, impaired judgment, and probable disorientation and confusion. Give examples of some of the simple one-step instructions that the person may be able to follow.
- Have regular emergency drills so that each member of the household has a specific task. Realize that the person with Alzheimer's disease cannot be expected to hold any responsibility in the crisis plan and that someone will need to take primary responsibility for supervising the individual.
- Always have at least an extra week's supply of any medical or personal hygiene items critical to the person's welfare, such as:
    - food and water
    - medications
    - incontinence undergarments
    - hearing aid batteries
- Keep an extra pair of the person's eyeglasses on hand.
- Be sure that the person with Alzheimer's wears an identification bracelet stating "memory loss" should he or she become lost or disoriented during the crisis. Contact your local Alzheimer's Association chapter and enroll the person in the Safe Return program.

- Under no circumstances should a person with Alzheimer's be left alone following a natural disaster. Do not count on the individual to stay in one place while you go to get help. Provide plenty of reassurance.

Who Would Take Care of the Person with Alzheimer's If Something Happened to You?

It is important to have a plan in case of your own illness, disability, or death.

- Consult a lawyer about setting up a living trust, durable power of attorney for health care and finances, and other estate planning tools.
- Consult with family and close friends to decide who will take responsibility for the person with Alzheimer's. You also may want to seek information about your local public guardian's office, mental health conservator's office, adult protective services, or other case management services. These organizations may have programs to assist the person with Alzheimer's in your absence.
- Maintain a notebook for the responsible person who will assume caregiving. Such a notebook should contain the following information:
    - emergency phone numbers
    - current problem behaviors and possible solutions
    - ways to calm the person with Alzheimer's
    - assistance needed with toileting, feeding, or grooming
    - favorite activities and foods
- Preview board and care or long-term care facilities in your community and select a few as possibilities. Share this information with the responsible person. If the person with Alzheimer's disease is no longer able to live at home, the responsible person will be better able to carry out your wishes for long-term care.

Conclusion

Home safety takes many forms. This chapter focuses on the physical environment and specific safety concerns. But the home environment also involves the needs, feelings, and lifestyles of you the caregiver, your family, and the person with Alzheimer's disease. Disability affects all family members, and it is crucial to maintain your emotional and physical welfare in addition to ensuring a safe environment.

We encourage you to make sure you have quiet time, time out, and time to take part in something you enjoy. Protect your own emotional and physical health. Your local Alzheimer's Association chapter can help you with the support and information you may need as you address this very significant checkpoint in your home safety list. You are extremely valuable. As you take on a commitment to care for a person with Alzheimer's, please take on the equally important commitment to care for yourself.

Additional Resources

Several organizations offer caregivers information about Alzheimer's disease. To learn more about support groups, services, research, and additional publications, you may wish to contact the following groups:

Alzheimer's Disease Education and Referral (ADEAR) Center
P.O. Box 8250
Silver Spring, MD 20907-8250
1-800-438-4380 (toll-free)
www.nia.nih.gov/alzheimers

The National Institute on Aging's ADEAR Center offers information and publications for families, caregivers, and professionals on diagnosis, treatment, patient care, caregiver needs, long-term care, education and training, and research related to Alzheimer's disease. Staff members answer telephone, email, and written requests and make referrals to local and national resources. The ADEAR website offers free, online publications in English and Spanish; email alert and online *Connections* newsletter subscriptions; an Alzheimer's disease clinical trials database; and more.

Alzheimer's Association
225 North Michigan Avenue, Floor 17
Chicago, IL 60601-7633
1-800-272-3900 (toll-free)
1-866-403-3073 (TDD/toll-free)
www.alz.org

The Alzheimer's Association is a national nonprofit association with a network of local chapters that provide education and support for people diagnosed with Alzheimer's disease, their families, and caregivers. The Association also supports research on Alzheimer's.

Alzheimer's Foundation of America
322 Eighth Avenue, 7th Floor
New York, NY 10001
1-866-232-8484 (toll-free)
www.alzfdn.org

The Alzheimer's Foundation of America provides care and services to individuals confronting dementia and to their caregivers and families through member organizations dedicated to improving quality of life. Services include a toll-free hotline, consumer publications and other educational materials, and conferences and workshops.

American Red Cross
2025 E Street, NW
Washington, DC 20006
1-800-733-2767
www.redcross.org

The Red Cross offers health information, health services, disaster relief, and emergency services to the public. Local chapters provide programs for older people, including safety courses and home nurse care instruction.

Eldercare Locator
1-800-677-1116 (toll-free)
www.eldercare.gov

Eldercare Locator is a nationwide directory-assistance service helping older people and their caregivers locate local support and resources. It is funded by the U.S. Administration on Aging, whose website at *www.aoa.gov* also features Alzheimer's information for families, caregivers, and healthcare professionals.

Family Caregiver Alliance
785 Market Street, Suite 750
San Francisco, CA 94103
1-800-445-8106 (toll-free)
www.caregiver.org

The Family Caregiver Alliance is a nonprofit organization that offers support services and information for people caring for adults with Alzheimer's, stroke, traumatic brain injuries, and other cognitive disorders.

Well Spouse Association
63 West Main Street, Suite H
Freehold, NJ 07728
1-800-838-0879 (toll-free)
www.wellspouse.org

This nonprofit organization gives support to spouses and partners of people who are chronically ill and/or disabled. It offers support groups and a newsletter.

INDEX

A

B

C

D

E

P

Q

R

S

T

U

V

W

X

Y

Z